# The US Healthcare Dilemma

# The US Healthcare Dilemma

## Mirrors and Chains

Michael T. McGuire
and William H. Anderson

**AUBURN HOUSE**
Westport, Connecticut • London

**Library of Congress Cataloging-in-Publication Data**

McGuire, Michael T., 1929–
    The US healthcare dilemma : mirrors and chains / Michael T.
McGuire and William H. Anderson.
      p.  cm.
    Includes bibliographical references and index.
    ISBN 0–86569–275–0 (alk. paper)
    1. Medical policy—United States.  2. Medical care—United States.
3. Medical economics—United States.  I. Anderson, William H.
(William Henry), 1940– .  II. Title.
    RA395.A3M39  1999
    362.1'0973—dc21       98–47752

British Library Cataloguing in Publication Data is available.

Library of Congress Catalog Card Number: 98–47752
ISBN: 0–86569–275–0

First published in 1999

Auburn House, 88 Post Road West, Westport, CT 06881
An imprint of Greenwood Publishing Group, Inc.
www.greenwood.com

Printed in the United States of America

The paper used in this book complies with the
Permanent Paper Standard issued by the National
Information Standards Organization (Z39.48–1984).

10 9 8 7 6 5 4 3 2 1

*To all US citizens who have
attempted to improve the quality of healthcare.*

# Contents

*Part I*

# Setting the Perspective

*Chapter 1*

# Ten Postulates

A better healthcare system is possible in the United States now. To satisfy our demands for quality, choice, accessibility, and economy, it is necessary to return to the concept of paying for what we get. There are ways to do this that are well within our reach—as communities and as a nation. In the chapters that follow we do three things. We critically examine obsolete assumptions and practices that have intruded into, and come to dominate, our thinking about healthcare solutions. We document what needs to be done next. And we expand on the following ten postulates:

- The "right" to healthcare is not a helpful concept, because it cannot be defined in an operational way. Debate over it serves only to cloud our minds as we search for practical healthcare solutions.

- Medical care is not a fungible commodity, measurable in equal units. Even in principle, it cannot be allocated to everyone in an equal way.

- Healthcare is a transaction between individual patients and professional providers. Corporate and governmental insurers are ancillary participants.

- Incentives are more effective modifiers of behavior than rules.

- People would rather cooperate than be contentious, as long as the group performing the task is the right size.

- Dissatisfaction with diminished access to standard care has caused increased interest in largely ineffective "alternative" treatments.

- Growth of technology does not need to cause increases in costs. With proper incentives, costs will decrease while quality and access improve.

- The root cause of dissatisfaction with the current US healthcare system is over-reliance on insurance.

- Insurance does not make healthcare more affordable. It increases costs and often decreases quality and ease of access.
- A large proportion of healthcare costs occurs in the last year of life. That is how it should be. That is when we are sick.

*Chapter 2*

# The Setting, the Issues, the Questions

I spend at least four hours a week dealing with HMOs, hospitals, doctors, and the like . . . they all have a different story, play a different game, and often simply lie . . . No one in my family has a serious illness—just routine things with the kids . . . You have to wonder if they know what they are doing—on second thought you don't have to wonder. . . . To make matters worse, they change their rules every week . . . and do they inform me? You can guess the answer—months after the fact . . . American medicine is a mess. It's ill managed . . . it's greedy . . . and it's my family that is suffering . . . Cash and insurance policies don't make any difference . . . It's the system—better, it's the lack of a system that has made patients the victims of incompetence.

> Interview with a 38-year-old married mother of three children,
> Ivy League graduate, and CEO of a thriving company

## INTRODUCTION

On several things we can all agree. We want quality healthcare. We want it at a reasonable cost. And we want easy access to healthcare professionals.

So why are we having so much difficulty getting what we all want? Why is healthcare so unevenly distributed? Why is it so difficult to arrange an appointment with a physician on short notice? Why are there such great discrepancies in the quality of healthcare providers? Why are so many patients complaining about poor healthcare quality? Why does the cost of healthcare continually rise? Why are there so many malpractice cases? Why are some healthcare executives reaping tremendous financial profits while some patients go untreated? Why are the federal and state legislatures so disorganized in their attempts to regulate healthcare and why are they continually changing their commitments to healthcare? Why is the number of patient- and disease-oriented advocacy groups on the rise?

*In short, why can't we or why won't we solve our healthcare problems?*

There are many answers to these questions. Some are straightforward, some are not straightforward, and some can't be answered. This book is about some but not all of the answers. It is about the consequences that develop when systems are built on obsolete assumptions, when many of the incentives for providing healthcare are perverse, and when there are too many players in the healthcare arena. It is a book about the fact that neither the free market nor the government can satisfactorily solve our healthcare problems and why we have a five-decade history of fits and starts without any truly satisfactory healthcare solutions. It is a book about the fact that attempts to provide solutions to critical healthcare problems have overlooked essential features of human nature. Until these features are understood and incorporated into healthcare planning, expect more of the status quo—that is, brace yourself for continual change among healthcare payers, healthcare providers, and increasing dissatisfaction among healthcare recipients.

## THE 1950s

But we are ahead of ourselves. For the moment, let us step back in time and pick up the healthcare story when medical delivery in the United States was largely in the hands of patients, physicians, nurses, and hospitals. The year 1950 is a convenient date, for it was at this time that events which would contribute to and shape today's healthcare began to take place.

For those readers who are 60 or more years old, the events they probably remember best concern technological change. During the 1950s, technological advances began to improve the precision of medical diagnosis and treatment. Disease was in retreat. Patients became healthier and began to live longer. Optimism was the mood of the day. As a nation, we began to believe that we could cure cancer, diabetes, and schizophrenia. Young, idealistic medical and nursing students flocked to training schools to participate in what promised to be a society largely free of disease.

For readers who were born after 1950, it may be difficult to imagine the social impact of that optimism. The United States thought and felt differently than it does today. There were common goals for which Americans strived. People worked harder. They cooperated more. Their efforts were more directed and more productive. Distant social goals were in focus, and improving the nation's health was one of the more worthy and attractive goals. To speed things along, government and industry provided medical centers with funds for new and expensive equipment to carry out studies that two decades earlier would have been impossible to imagine.

In retrospect, it is easy enough to understand how optimism captured the day. Optimism is fun and especially so in a resource-affluent environment. Yet, in the shadows of our enthusiasm, little noticed but critically important changes began to occur. As America entered the 1960s, many Americans failed to notice the gradually rising costs of healthcare, just as they failed to appreciate that diagnosis and treatment were becoming increasingly dependent on technology. Nor did they notice that it became harder to find the proverbial country doctor or the urban general practitioner.[1] Medical specialties had become the career objectives of most young physicians as the nation's medical schools churned out thousands of surgeons, internists, and psychiatrists.

With increasing numbers of doctors turning to specialties, medicine's financial picture began to change. No longer did the average physician have to carry a full workload to make financial ends meet. Suddenly, there was the possibility of a large income, and even wealth. These changes were not without their consequences, and for healthcare the consequences are clear. Medicine's heart began to decouple from its past traditions, in particular its sense of social purpose. What had once been primarily a service profession began to look more and more like a business.

## HEALTH INSURANCE

The 1950s were also the period in which insurance began to exert its influence over the direction and quality of healthcare. Historically, the origins of health insurance can be traced back to World War II and wage-price controls. In the early 1940s, there was a serious shortage of skilled workers. As corporations competed for the few available and talented individuals that were not in the armed services, they found that by adding insurance benefits they could achieve a competitive advantage yet still comply with wage-price regulations.

At first, health insurance was sensible because it was limited primarily to unexpected illnesses and catastrophic losses. With time, however, the scope of coverage expanded; and by the mid-1970s, insurance companies were paying not only for unexpected illnesses, but also for such expected events as pregnancies, childrens' earaches, and poison oak. With these changes, insurance coverage drifted away from its long-established and well-tested principle that it offers a defense against rare events. As the drift continued, insurance companies discovered that they had become the financial *deep pockets* for everything from minor cuts to the removal of brain tumors.

Consequences followed which even deep pockets could not avoid. For healthcare, the most important of these was the loss of market discipline that develops when one uses one's own money, not someone else's, to pay for what one receives. Nor, with time, would the loss of market discipline change. Loss of market discipline has remained a thorn in the side of literally every attempt to devise and implement an equitable solution to the problems that plague our healthcare system.

Again, many readers may be too young to have experienced medicine without insurance, which was largely the case before the 1950s. Moreover, given that today health insurance is so commonplace, its purveyors so aggressive, and its propaganda so prevalent, the thought of not having health insurance is likely to frighten even the healthiest and richest of individuals. Yet, for a moment, consider the sequence of events that characterizes the history of many health insurance companies. (1) A company decides to enter the health insurance field. (2) It offers complete or near complete health coverage at attractive rates. (3) Individuals and companies purchase the insurance. (4) Claims begin to add up. (5) After a period, the company finds that its claims cost more that the expected 40 to 50 cents of every dollar collected and that it is not achieving its projected profit target. (6) The company then begins to alter its policies by restricting its coverage and introducing payment constraints such as coverage deductibles and co-payment schemes. (7) With profits still not meeting expectations, the company begins to cap the frequency with which patients can visit healthcare providers and increasingly places restrictions on treatments. (8) At this point, those who are insured begin to spend increasing amounts of time trying to arrange appointments with their providers, filling in insurance company forms, and waiting to have their claims processed. (9) Next, restrictions, such as requiring healthcare providers to obtain insurance company approval for treatments, are imposed.[2] (10) Next, payments to providers are capped regardless of the time required to provide services. (11) Finally, after enough frustration, the company discontinues its healthcare lines, sells its healthcare unit to another company, or increases its premiums to a level that only the rich can afford.

The preceding scenario might suggest that insurance companies are malicious entities as well as the primary culprits responsible for many of the current US healthcare predicaments. This is only partially true. To their credit, insurance companies acknowledge their desire to make a profit. To their discredit, making a profit is ultimately more important than carrying out their contractual commitments.[3] The desire for profit is not the only factor, however. Poor insurance judgments and overzealous clients can add to a company's problems.

Poor insurance judgments are those in which companies fail to estimate accurately the number and the cost of claims for the individuals they insure. The fact that approximately 30% of healthcare payers overuse their insurance coverage only compounds the problem. Overutilization is analogous to having a contract with the local supermarket, which permits one to take anything one wants from the shelves for a fixed price each month. Suddenly, one's idea of dinner shifts from pasta or hamburger to a gourmet event bracketed by fine wine and liqueurs. The inflationary costs of day-to-day healthcare add yet further problems. Dissatisfied patients and lawyers have convinced many providers that one way to protect themselves from lawsuits is to engage in what might best be termed "defensive medicine," which equates with ordering an excessive number of tests and undertaking an excessive number of procedures.

We return to each of these points in later chapters. For the present, the key question to keep in mind is: *Do we want the kind of healthcare system we now have for ourselves, for our children, for our friends, and even for our enemies?*

## GOVERNMENT AND HEALTHCARE AS A "RIGHT"

To return to the 1950s, a few farsighted individuals voiced their concerns about where the "new medicine" was heading. As they did, Congress, state legislatures, federal and state funding agencies, pharmaceutical companies, universities, and the American Medical Association largely listened with deaf ears—optimism and unlimited resources have their own imperatives. Yet, like deep pockets, optimism and funding also have their limits. Eventually, reality asserts itself. For healthcare, nearly three decades would pass before the optimism and funding bubble would burst. True, during the period between the 1950s and the 1980s, many new cures for diseases were discovered and advances in our knowledge about the causes of diseases increased significantly. Yet it is also true that by the mid-1970s Medicare costs were rising at an alarming rate, as were malpractice costs, and patients and healthcare providers were becoming increasingly disenfranchised.

The 1950s also mark the beginning of a fundamental change in attitude about healthcare. Both government and healthcare recipients began to believe that healthcare is a *right*, not a privilege or something one pays for. In principle, the idea of healthcare as a right is attractive. Moreover, to the degree that it is a right, it makes perfect sense that the government should see to it that the right is respected and enforced. On the other hand, if healthcare is a privilege or something one pays for, we enter the marketplace. As most readers know, the United States has straddled the fence, hoping that the right–privilege conundrum would solve itself. Had it done so, this book would not have been written.

The basic problem with the idea that "healthcare is a right" is that its goals can not be achieved. Nonachievement is not simply due to a lack of effort by many healthcare providers or a shortage of money. The primary reasons lie elsewhere. People disagree about what should and should not be a right. They disagree about who should determine if rights are honored. Further, structures designed to implement rights are imperfect. Those with the responsibility of determining if rights are being honored use different evaluation criteria. In turn, disputes develop, and disputes are costly and time consuming. The failure to realize such limitations is a basic flaw in what otherwise is a commendable idea. Nevertheless, by the early 1990s the view that healthcare is a right had blossomed into a fully articulated political philosophy, supported by a cadre of well-intentioned idealists and politicians whose knowledge of disease and healthcare delivery often appeared to be acquired more from reruns of *Dr. Kildare* (a 1950s TV program about an idealistic doctor) than either fact or experience.

The United States is a democratic country and nothing of major social importance usually happens rapidly except declarations of war, as in the days following Pearl Harbor or Operation Desert Storm. Typically, problems arise, and there are fits and starts at solving them. In the early stages, little is usually solved. In the later stages, problems may be impossible to solve, largely because multiple players have entered the problem arena and insist that they must be part of the solution. The history of agricultural supports (farmers receiving money not to grow things), much of welfare, and illegal immigration are familiar examples.

And thus what was anticipated by a few in the 1950s would come to pass with healthcare in the 1980s and 1990s.[4] By the mid-1980s, Medicare and Medicaid were out of control for many of the same reasons that health insurance coverage was out of control.[5] Concurrently, instances of medical fraud were increasing, a sure sign that medicine had lost its bearings and greed rather than service had become the modus oporandi for many of its practitioners.[6] HMOs began to expand like a new virus for which the marketplace's immune system had not yet developed a resistance. By the early 1990s, government began to bail out of healthcare. Congressional cuts in Medicare reduced the federal government's responsibility for healthcare payments and left the treatment of many of the poor and indigent to the states, churches, and others to solve.[7] President Clinton's efforts to develop a national healthcare system were shipwrecked before they left dry dock. Yet, many HMOs and insurance companies continued to flourish despite the fact that somewhere between 40 and 50% of the healthcare insurance dollar went for administration, CEO salaries, and investor profit.[8] By 1998, the majority of Americans depended on some type of insurance policy or HMO to pay part to all of their healthcare costs; they too had become players in the marketplace.

## MARKETPLACE AND GOVERNMENT SOLUTIONS

Do not be fooled by the idea that all problems can be solved if they are allowed to play out in the marketplace. Although there are many virtues to a marketplace economy, the marketplace means that players are trying to have it their way. What is often forgotten about the marketplace is that individuals and corporations are self-interested; they will attempt to make a profit at others' expense, and a percentage of free-market players will fail.[9]

Of course one can argue that, if left to its own devices, the free market could lead eventually to an optimal healthcare system. While there is no evidence to disprove this possibility, it is unlikely to be tested in the United States. The system under which we operate is far from a free market. Competition among healthcare providers is impeded both by loss of price sensitivity from insurance and by a regulatory environment that favors large-scale operations with their associated swarms of providers, administrators, auditors, and lawyers. Loss of direction is an inevitable outcome. Hospitals close because their bills are not paid, and irrespective of obvious need, patients are often denied treatment because persons other than healthcare providers (e.g. administrators) have decided that treatment costs too much. In such an environment it is not surprising that hands-on providers and hospitals often pad bills and charge for treatments they have not provided.[10] As these events swirl about us, quality healthcare has become harder to find.

If the marketplace can not guarantee an acceptable healthcare solution, what about government? Don't be led astray by the government either. The US government does an excellent job at many things, such as building and training armed forces, nudging states to follow federal laws, and developing bureaucracies. State and county governments can also be effective in certain areas. But government also fails at many things, such as delivering the mail, fighting drug use, being honest, allocating resources according to equitable principles, and resisting the temptations offered by special interests. In short, the government has yet to prove that it can be an effective catalyst in providing quality healthcare solutions.

## WHERE DOES ONE TURN?

Where does one turn? Our answer is to identify those obsolete assumptions that guide our current healthcare system and thinking, and to reintroduce fundamental features of human behavior into healthcare policy. Reintroducing features of human behavior means taking a close look at human motivations, how human beings organize and regulate themselves, how they develop reciprocal relationships, how they act to reduce uncertainty, and how they address and solve problems that must address the fact that individuals differ. Left to their own devices, humans organize themselves in small groups. They invest primarily in kin and in nonkin with whom they have developed reciprocal relationships. They develop close, intermediate, and distant friends, and the degree of trust and reciprocity differs at each distance. They develop their own rules of behavior. They communicate what is important to one another. They help one another, and they ostracize those who refuse to help. And they do all of this without governmental help and administration, taxation, oversight committees, and the like. But more about these points presently.

## CONCLUDING COMMENTS

The two remaining chapters in Part I develop our perspective towards healthcare by discussing healthcare myths and the present state of US healthcare. Part II focuses on what the key healthcare players—patients, healthcare providers, and healthcare payers—want. Part III discusses key missing elements in today's planning for healthcare. Part IV discusses viable options for our healthcare crisis and finishes with a chapter devoted to questions and answers.

## NOTES

1. It is of interest that this problem has not improved, and that it remains refractory to regulatory efforts. See, for example, R. A. Rosenblatt and J. Hook, *Los Angeles Times*, 13 June 1997, in which they analyze a bill in the US House of Representatives that would shift Medicare dollars from urban to rural HMOs.

2. Mental health treatment is usually the first casualty. See the work of A. E. Lansing and colleagues in *General Hospital Psychiatry* 19 (1997): 112–118. Managed care systems have a strong tendency to limit psychiatric hospital admissions to those patients who are imminently homicidal, suicidal, or unable to provide for their basic needs.

3. Regulations and government mandates appear to be a clumsy tool in the service of resource allocation. See G. Anders and L. McGinley, *Wall Street Journal*, 6 March 1997. They document how elderly patients are becoming economic jackpots for homecare companies due to open-ended reimbursement by Medicare.

4. The unthinkable has become at least plausible. Consider, for example, the report by G. Kolata in the *New York Times*, 13 April 1997. A Cleveland prosecutor has accused a local medical center of seeking to hasten the deaths of terminally ill patients in order to obtain their organs for transplant.

5. This problem is at least being recognized by certain elements of the political elite. For example, R. A. Rosenblatt and E. Chen, *Los Angeles Times*, 25 April 1997, report estimates that the Medicare hospital trust fund will be insolvent in four years.

6. As third-party payers change their policies, so do the providers change their emphasis. A. Sharp, *Wall Street Journal*, 1 May 1997, reports on the tendency of doctors and hospitals to chase pregnant women on Medicaid, who have become the most lucrative patients in the healthcare business.

7. A bill introduced into the US Senate would expect the wealthy to pay higher fees under the Medicare program. See the report of R. A. Rosenblatt, *Los Angeles Times*, 25 June 1997.

8. On the other hand, patients are not without legal recourse. D. R. Olmos reports in *Los Angeles Times*, 11 July 1997, of agreements to settle claims of patients against healthcare executives.

9. Sometimes they fail in spectacular ways. See the report of A. C. Adams, *Wall Street Journal*, 20 June 1997, for a review of management problems, including stock irregularities, accounting curiosities, bickering boards, and CEO musical chairs.

10. Fraud is part of the human condition, but some regulatory environments are

more conducive to it than others. See, for example, G. Anders and L. McGinley, *Wall Street Journal*, 6 May 1997. Enforcement budgets are on the rise as government agencies are training their sights on big, complex cases. The FBI now has 350 people investigating the healthcare industry, up by 290 from October 1996.

*Chapter 3*

# Healthcare Myths and Misunderstandings

It's 4:30 . . . I've been here since 9:00 A.M., and all I saw was a nurse . . . I don't think that is right. . . . I pay taxes. I work. I raise my kids. But I can't pay for the costs of health insurance and still feed my children. . . . I came here today because my boy has an earache . . . I don't think that he should have to wait seven hours for treatment when he is crying all the time.

> Discussion with a 47-year-old mother of two
> children after leaving a public hospital clinic

## INTRODUCTION

Myths and misunderstanding are at the center of many of the seemingly unsolvable problems of healthcare. What are these myths and misunderstandings?

In what ways do they constrain and delay equitable solutions to healthcare? These questions are addressed in this chapter. Yet even to begin to answer them requires some homework. Perhaps the best place to begin is with a discussion about two contrasting ways of interpreting experience.

## ORGANIZING AND EXPLAINING EXPERIENCE

The history of human thought has been marked by competition between two distinct and contradictory ways of organizing and explaining experience. The first dates back centuries. The second is of more recent origin.

"Faith-and-authority" is the name we will give to the first way. A concept is considered to be true to the extent that it is enunciated by individuals of high status and leadership. Since prehistoric times, this pre-scientific method has been overwhelming in its influence. There are good reasons why this is so. Faith-and-authority is a highly efficient means of transferring information about the solutions to old problems. The concept finds its greatest utility in pre-literate societies, which aspire to the preservation of proven survival strategies. In particular, it must have been useful during the long period of human evolution known to biologists as the "environment of evolutionary adaptation," when our main problems were finding food and avoiding predators. A chief's authoritative declaration of the strategy that had served his predecessors well was usually sufficient.

Faith-and-authority is an excellent method for preserving satisfactory (but seldom optimal) solutions to familiar problems; in effect, a conservative strategy, one with the admonition to "go with what works, and not get fancy." A typical day in the lives of our prehistoric ancestors illustrates this point. We are walking through the tropical savanna, working to make a living. Among other problems, this task requires remembering the locations of edible plant concentrations and remaining vigilant for attacks by competing groups and animals. When competitor or animal threats are detected, the chief orders appropriate evasive action. Action is taken and, in most instances, the members of the group survive. When survival occurs, decision by authority is highly adaptive.

There are of course other ways that members of the group might behave. For instance, suppose that a predator is detected. Rather than fleeing, a member of the group decides to disregard the admonitions of the chief and observe the predator and to investigate the predator's behavior. The decision to observe might have two outcomes. One is that the individual will forfeit his contribution to the gene pool of the next generation. The other is that he might gain new knowledge and increase his survival chances in the future.

Faith-and-authority has its place and most of us accept its value, as in instances when a mother warns her child not to approach a hot stove. Faith-and-authority is also a highly useful strategy for promoting group cohesion. As was the case with our distant relatives (and is the case with other terrestrial primates), core organizing principles of *Homo sapiens* include the formation and perpetuation of kinship groups, the development of hierarchies within groups, the maintenance of hierarchies with dominance and deference signals, and the defense of territories from stranger groups through marking and threat display behavior. In these activities, both the assertion of authority and deference to it are not only critical, but they also serve to enhance group solidarity and preserve collections of useful experience. Further, when these core-organizing principles are the bases of groups, socially useful events usually follow. For example, groups tend to develop stable social structures. Interlocking alliances are formed in which the members share assumptions about how to solve important problems of group cohesion and survival. Consensus is achieved on how to deal with new challenges, and social friction is minimized.

This is not to say that faith-and-authority is without its problems or critics. As a way of understanding and explaining the world, the precept does not always converge on the truth. In addition, the idea often fails when it comes to solving new and critically important problems or in optimizing solutions to old problems. Knowledge is not necessarily progressive. Rather, it follows, for good or ill, the trajectory of cultural evolution and, in part, reflects the biases of leaders. Moreover, when the positive features of this type of thinking are peeled away, a fundamental shortcoming is apparent—one known to classical logicians as the *ad baculum* argument, or the idea that "I win a debate because of my authority or power."

Opposed to the mode of faith-and-authority is that of "observation-and-logic." This is the scientific method. This way of thinking is relatively new. It made its first appearance in ancient Greece, but only since the Enlightenment has it received wide acceptance. In this mode of thought, doubt reigns and conclusions are always provisional, awaiting the emergence of new information. Explanatory hypotheses are tested and supported or rejected by experiment. No idea is ever shown perfectly valid for all time. Rather, understanding and explanation are matters of progressive approximation.

Observation-and-logic is not without its own set of limitations. Findings that conflict with cherished beliefs are often met in the social and political communities with derision. This is usually the case when one reports findings that an admired leader is corrupt. (There is an Indian proverb to the effect that one who is about to tell the truth should have one foot in the stirrup.) To advance knowledge—that is, to assert that our understanding and explanations of the world are different from what they are thought to be—is often to be in the minority. And this can be dangerous. On this point, one has only to recall the disbelief and negative responses to the initial documentation that many of our industrial products were actively depleting the ozone layer of the earth.

Decades ago, the sociologist Max Weber addressed the issue of new knowledge in his discussion of the "fact/value dichotomy." He noted that some of us view the world as if facts are distinct and knowable in themselves, and independent of human agency, while others behave as if facts are nothing unless congruent with wishes or values (in other words, if we want something to be true badly enough, we will think it so). That this value approach to truth is ever present has been recently suggested by an erstwhile White House staff member who was quoted as saying that "Truth is whatever you want it to be."

A convenient example illustrating what Weber had in mind is found in the work of the Soviet biologist Trofim Lysenko. With Stalin's enthusiastic approval, Lysenko asserted that learned characteristics, such as the ability to solve complex mathematical problems, could be inherited. This assertion implies that skills that are learned somehow work their way into our genes, and in turn through the process of genetic transmission, the acquired traits appear in future generations. Although experiments repeatedly established that Lysenko's conjecture was false, not only was it widely embraced among agriculturists in the Soviet Union for over two decades, but those who practiced agriculture using Lysenko's ideas consistently had poor agricultural yields.

What has all this philosophy to do with healthcare? In human political decisions, and especially in the emotion-laden realms of life and death and pain and loss, we are especially vulnerable to poorly formed arguments that pander to our hopes and wishes. In particular, we avoid the often dreary facts we must face to move our system of healthcare toward rational solutions. Being human, our efforts at developing rational solutions will be flawed and incomplete. Yet as a starting point, it is critical to remind ourselves that there are facts about healthcare that can be identified and that will not go away. We ignore them at the peril of failure. In addition, to the degree that we address these facts, we will see that much of what passes for public debate has been based on myth or misunderstanding. Let us consider them.

## RIGHTS AND RESPONSIBILITIES

Let us return to the idea that healthcare is a "right," for it is a convenient place to begin our inquiry into healthcare myths and misunderstanding. Pollsters often ask the question, "Is healthcare a right?" Most people answer as if the question had a rational response. Yet it does not. Moreover, when the question is examined closely, answers turn out to be tangles of contradictions, not as clearly or easily formulated as one might suppose. This seemingly clear and straightforward question cannot be answered without separating facts and values.

The concept of rights grew out of the flowering of individual freedom during the Enlightenment. Thomas Jefferson in the Declaration of Independence expressed the concept with great eloquence. In essence, rights are conditions that naturally adhere to individuals as a result of God's creation. Self-autonomy is good example, because it is an inherently human characteristic and thus may be considered a right. Rights are not gifts, awards, or "entitlements." Governments have no capacity to confer them. Rather, governments can only secure them at the collective will of a sovereign citizenry. Further, rights are not processes, nor can they be defined quantitatively. Instead, they are operational expressions of the freedom to be unmolested and to act in a morally sound way without coercion.

Rights have no meaning without responsibilities. Indeed, rights and responsibilities connect to each other as surely as do the subject and predicate of a sentence. In the tradition of the Enlightenment, we enjoy rights as a condition of our humanity. Properly understood, rights reside equally to all humanity. They are not some sort of beneficent currency that can be given to an individual or demographically defined group. They carry the positive obligation to conduct ourselves with integrity and social responsibility.

When politicians seek to award a "right," they mean to use the power of the state to transfer value from one group to another group under the umbrella of a legal statute. Thus when such a "right" is awarded to one person, it simultaneously implies or incurs an obligation on someone else to provide the value that is transferred. This is what happens, for example, with our income tax system, which is based on the concept that those who have more money should pay a different tax than those who have less money. A better term, as well as one that preserves the clarity of the meaning of a right in its historical context, is "entitlement"—grants of value from one group to another through the intermediation of government. Applied to healthcare, it seems clear that whatever else it might be, healthcare is not a right. It is not something conferred upon us because of our humanity. It is something that we do for each other. If it is not a right, can it be an "entitlement?"

Entitlement, or value conferred without corresponding obligation, may be a morally dubious concept, but in principle conferring value without associated obligation should be possible if the value received is measurable and it has clear boundaries. Without these conditions, chaos is likely to reign if only because the donors and recipients have unavoidable incentives to disagree as to the quantity and quality of the entitlement.

As an example, consider the possibility of a citizenry receiving entitlement to housing without corresponding obligation. At first glance, it seems plausible that the government might guarantee housing to all its citizens. Yet, such guarantees are meaningless unless the citizenry has the resources available to exercise the entitlement. (If resources were available, there would be no need for the entitlement. This is the case, for example with the oxygen we breathe. It is an abundant resource available to all and there is no associated entitlement.) Thus, a reasonable assumption is that some citizens lack adequate resources, and it is these individuals to which the entitlement is directed primarily. Even here, however, a closer look reveals that the concept of entitlement is inherently unstable. Housing may be as humble as a tent or as splendid as a palace. Given this wide spectrum of housing possibilities, it is unlikely that a consensus can be reached between those that provide or enforce the housing entitlement and its recipients concerning what people "want" and what they believe they "need" with respect to housing. Those who provide housing (e.g., the government, a corporation) are likely to see wants and needs differently from the recipients of housing. The potential discrepancy between "want" and "need" does not end here, however. Related issues are likely to arise. Does this housing entitlement then include furnishing? If so, how much and what kind? Do the recipients have a choice? If not, why not? How much land should surround the house? Does the dweller exercise ownership rights over this land? Is there entitlement to an oriental rug, or how about two? Or what if a person doesn't like oriental rugs? In short, an entitlement to housing is problematic at best, and worst of all, by accepting the entitlement, recipients also accept the fact that they relinquish control of many of the choices they might otherwise exercise.

Complex though it may seem, entitlement to housing is a trivial problem compared to entitlement for healthcare. At least housing is tangible. While parts of healthcare are also tangible, there are large elements of emotionally laden concerns such as kindness, courtesy, timeliness, pain relief, supportive relationships among family members, and finally, dealing with death. People who count themselves as free are unlikely to be satisfied to relinquish control over these vital areas of human concern, even if they are assured of the essentially benign intention of donors. We each own our own bodies. If we assign care of these bodies to a system of entitlement, we are saying that we expect the care more suitable for domestic animals—that is, well-meant, usually competent, but with few choices or much autonomy.

Healthcare is not a fungible commodity in which one unit or part may be substituted or exchanged for another unit or part. The siren song of entitlement to healthcare builds from the assumption that that some measurable quantity of care may be assigned arbitrarily to each of us, as if healthcare is a ration of grain, interchangeable, with each unit of measure identical to every other—"How many scoops for you?" Care, of course, is not like grain. Ideally, it resembles a custom-designed machine, or a work of art. If we had entitlement to works of art, what quality would these works be likely to have? Or if we had entitlement to housing, would we wish to live in the results of it?

Because healthcare is not a fungible commodity, it cannot be equally distributed. Some of us will refuse it, and others will insist on quite a lot. Some of us will need or want more of it than others, and some of us will be willing to do whatever it takes to fulfill this perceived need. Insisting that care be equally distributed merely ensures that other measures for exchange will occur, such as bribery, barter, blackmail, or political corruption. In effect, the rigid application of law and regulation to the healthcare system will suffer the same fate as attempts at price controls, which inevitably bring with them shortages of desirable services and surpluses of unpopular ones.

## INSURANCE AND AFFORDABILITY

A second misunderstanding or myth is the belief that insurance reduces the cost of healthcare. In fact, just the opposite is true. It not only increases the cost of medical care to all but a very few but it also makes healthcare less available to many. Failure to appreciate this fact is one of the most important causes of cloudy thinking about healthcare finance. To illustrate this point, try the following experiment. Ask a friend to imagine a world in which routine healthcare costs would be paid by out-of-pocket funds. The response, vigorous and immediate, is likely to be "I couldn't afford it." Yet, do not stop here. Pursue the matter. Explain that, in the aggregate, insurance inflates costs by inserting barriers, in time and space, between delivery of services and their payment. Point out that this causes price insensitivity, which leads to the loss of market discipline. Further explain that, at the very least, insurance introduces costs that are in the range from 40 to 50% of every dollar invested and which often are unnecessary or which go to stockholders and to managerial salaries. Ask again about paying for routine care directly. Your friend is likely to again mutter "I couldn't afford it" and walk away, eyes glazed over. As your friend walks away, remind him or her that you were talking about routine healthcare costs. Although the experiment may be disappointing, perhaps you have planted a seed in your friend's mind, one that will make him or her more responsive to alternative ways of financing healthcare in the future.

Let us return to the basics. The original function of insurance was to provide monetary compensation for losses brought about by bad luck, such as an unexpected injury or the destruction of one's property by fire. This function implies that the losses are not expected—that is, not routine—but that they are unusual or rare as well as associated with painful or dangerous personal or financial consequences when they occur. It is for these reasons that most of us purchase fire insurance for our homes. However, would it be reasonable to have insurance cover such routine activities such as purchasing the weekly groceries? If insurance companies were so foolish as to entertain this idea, what might be the trends of food quality, availability, and cost? Would insurance companies feel it necessary to introduce a concept of a "gatekeeper" at the supermarket entrance, as they now do for many healthcare treatments? Would a primary care nutritionist advise you that gruel is adequate for your needs, and that under no circumstances are you permitted to have potato chips? If you protest that you will be glad to pay for the chips yourself, would your counselor explain that this is not permitted either, because to allow a purchase outside the plan would mean promoting an unfavorable selection bias that would be unfair to others and increase costs?

When dealing with insurance companies it is always wise to ask, "Does the insurance company remember that it is your money they are using?" Rarely is the answer yes. Once the premium is paid, the majority of insurance companies act as if all the money is theirs. Moreover, if they were in the food insurance business, any actual food delivery would be termed something akin to "nutritional loss," to be minimized in the interests of maximizing executive salaries, shareholder value, and company longevity.

We understand intuitively that insurance for such routine purposes as purchasing groceries is a bad idea. Yet we often fail to appreciate that the same problems arise in healthcare funding. Much medical care is routine or elective in nature. *To use insurance as a funding mechanism for costs that we are certain to incur is guaranteed to increase costs while diminishing quality and availability.* On the other hand, some medical care is required unexpectedly, urgently, and necessarily. In our view, this is the proper kind of event to insure for and the proper place for reimbursement by an insurance program.

Insurance companies are legitimate businesses. They sell a service that it is often wise to buy. The service is that of risk sharing. They have a skill that allows them to provide this service and to make an overall profit. The skill is actuarial calculation. Insurance companies know, or they should know, the likelihood that your ship will sink or the likelihood that your arm will break. By means of actuarial calculation, they are able to know how much premium to charge to a pool of risk-bearers to assure payment of damages to the few and still emerge with a profit. When insurance companies begin to offer services outside this sphere of competence, all manner of mischief begins to occur, the most important of which is that they forget what business they are in, or should be in. Healthcare insurance companies, because they are being asked to pay for claims, assume, erroneously, that they know how to provide medical care and that they should be the final judges of just what care is appropriate. After all, it's their money.

We began this section by saying that healthcare insurance increases the costs of healthcare. Yet healthcare is not the only area in which attempted cost-sensitive solutions add significant unnecessary costs. Two sectors of the economy have suffered from cost increases quite out of proportion to reasonable expectation or inflation—healthcare and education. In both cases the underlying problem is the uncoupling of the time and place of payment from the time and place of service delivery. In the case of higher education, it is the easy availability of guaranteed federal loans. In the case of healthcare, it is largely the use of insurance for routine and expected events that has contributed to inflation. As a result, it has become a matter of bitter resignation in some quarters that healthcare costs are destined to rise forever and that some sort of dictatorial intervention is required. In subsequent chapters we will see why this scenario does not have to unfold, but grasping this insight requires that we face facts rather than wishes and conform our plans to some harmony with our human nature and our political traditions.

## FINDING THE HOLY GRAIL—COMMONLY PROPOSED SOLUTIONS

Acceptable solutions to the delivery of healthcare have eluded us for decades in spite of the attention of thoughtful experts. Analogies for the difficulty are easy to find. One that immediately comes to mind is that of the six blind men trying to describe an elephant. Captain Ahab's search for Moby Dick also seems fitting. That solutions have remained refractory to our best efforts suggests that we have yet to reach consensus on a set of underlying assumptions that should apply to healthcare. Only when consensus is reached can we proceed with the essential technical solutions. Failure in public problem solving is the likely outcome whenever we attempt to apply a solution that is not consistent with the political, economic, and cultural mores with which Americans generally agree. Currently, healthcare has imbedded itself within crosscurrents of mutually exclusive imperatives; for example, that everyone should receive equal care and yet also have the right to have robust choices available.

Let us consider some of the contradictions that exemplify these crosscurrents.

## Price Controls

Few things bring cheer more quickly to the heart of a politician than the elegant simplicity of price controls. In one form or another, every generation apparently needs to learn anew that fixing prices by law is the very essence of folly. In ancient Egypt, the pharaohs considered it only natural to mandate the proper ratio of the values of gold and silver. Within easy memory are the mile-long lines of cars awaiting fuel during the oil crisis of the 1970s. Most recently, the president and Congress have engaged in a festival of mutual congratulations as they "solved" the crisis of Medicare funding by the simple expedient of reducing the payments they allow to physicians and hospitals.

Economics and politics remain arcane sciences in many ways, and reasonable economists and politicians may differ in their theoretical approaches. Yet there is one thing they know with sublime certainty; namely, they understand how shortages and surpluses can be created. To create a shortage, simply pass a law requiring sellers to part with their goods for less money than they believe their goods are worth. For a surplus, insist that buyers pay more for goods than buyers believe is warranted. So simple, and so routinely ignored! The very essence of the consequences of Max Weber's fact/value dichotomy—Max would be amused. Cynics using this line of reasoning might argue that politicians know these facts, but they also know that the resultant chaos can be blamed on someone or something else, while they remain champions in giving the people what they want or believe they deserve.

## Government-Directed Programs

Critics of our current mechanism of healthcare delivery most often offer some variant of government medicine as an improved alternative, pointing to the fact that government-directed programs are the solution embraced by most other advanced countries. That one or another of these programs has not been adopted in the United States is taken as evidence that powerful impediments exist. Yet a close examination of these supposed impediments usually reveals that at heart they are value conflicts—we cherish many things as much as we cherish healthcare. Perhaps the most obvious example has to do with our political culture, in which the United States differs from most other advanced countries. We really believe at a basic level in the ideas embodied in the Declaration of Independence and in the qualities of character that support them, such as individual responsibility, self-reliance, and the expectation of limited government.[1] Our sister democracies in Britain, France, Germany, Canada, and elsewhere do not share this perspective. Popular sovereignty is not part of their political landscape. In Britain, for example, and even in Canada, the people are, at heart, still subjects of the Crown. Moreover, in Britain, no written constitution limits the areas of life into which the power of government may extend. A core assumption of political life is that government may do anything, provided that a majority in Parliament acquiesce. Are we ready to sacrifice our freedom and allow government to manage our healthcare system? We believe not.

Those who advocate government-directed healthcare are not easily dissuaded from their views. Does not military medicine work? they ask. Or if the military model is not suitable, what about healthcare in Canada?

The US government provides a comprehensive system of medical care for members of the armed services and their families. There are some problems with this system of delivery, but generally speaking, the quality and accessibility are good. So why not extend it to a civilian venue? One answer is that cost would be problematic. But the cost point aside, the key issue is that the culture of military service is not comparable with that of civilian life. Military personnel do as they are told. They subordinate individual autonomy in the service of the common mission. That is their core value. They are willing to risk their lives at the order of the president. Civilians are not (and should not be) willing to do that, absent an extraordinary national danger. Put another way, a nation that accepts military medicine for civilians would not be a free society. It would have to agree to accept the fact that medicine would be available as the government decided it should be available.

Then there is the case for adopting the Canadian model. The United States, it is said, should emulate the system currently in place to our north. There, healthcare personnel work for the government, which maintains the system by tax revenue. Most Canadians, most of the time, are satisfied with the services provided, although in recent times there have been notable increases in the waiting times for elective procedures as well as procedures that are not so elective. There are at least three concerns that cast doubt on the suitability of the Canadian model for the United States. The first we have noted. The Canadian political culture is more tolerant of paternalistic government than that of the United States. Second, the Canadian healthcare experience is ameliorated by the presence of a more free-market approach in its southern neighbor, with most Canadians living close enough to the border to access care not available through their government system. The Canadian system works as well as it does, at least to some extent, because the United States provides an occasionally useful alternative. Finally, Canada, in common with much of the rest of the industrialized world, does not have the entrepreneurial incentives in the healthcare arena that stimulate innovative techniques, many of which contribute to medical progress worldwide. On the latter point, and allowing that costs remain a serious healthcare concern in the United States, few of us are likely to be eager to halt the advance of new technologies. If you doubt this point, ask yourself which of the drugs and advanced surgical techniques you would be ready to abandon.

### Insurance-Based Solutions

We have already discussed some of the limitations of insurance-based solutions to healthcare. More needs to be said, however. From one perspective, the utility of insurance has stood the test of time, and reimbursing clients for losses arising from unexpected misfortune is the primary reason for its its longevity. However, as we have noted, both unintended and undesirable consequences follow from attempts to fund routine and commonplace healthcare expenses using an insurance model. As soon as patients succumb to the assumption that all or nearly all healthcare costs must be borne by insurance, and that this is the only way that the costs can be afforded, they become hostages to the profit motives of corporate policy. Because most individuals don't like being hostages, it might be assumed that there would be a rebellion against the insurance solution to healthcare. Pockets of rebellion sometimes appear, but on balance there is minimal direct opposition to insurance companies. Rather than question whether insurance can provide a viable healthcare solution, the tendency is to move the argument to the political sector. Disgruntled patients and clients ask for government regulations to save them from what they see as a corporate failure to apply human values in an area in which they are of primary importance.

To give the devil his due, insurance companies might properly argue that the bargain they offer is not unfair. They don't promise clients that all subsequent wishes will be fulfilled. They promise healthcare. Of course insurance companies have to reserve for themselves the right to define the limits of healthcare, otherwise their clients might decide that almost anything could be included under cover of an ever-enlarging healthcare umbrella. Thus begins ever-escalating arguments about what should be covered. Not surprisingly, insurance companies insist on narrow definitions of claims, regardless of the effectiveness of such definitions.[2] From the profit perspective, a cheap, ineffective treatment may be preferable to an expensive but effective one. Patients, on the other hand, insist that any treatment, or anything which purports to be a treatment, must be covered either in full or nearly in full, quite without regard to any calculus of cost-effectiveness. "If I want it, I should get it, because, after all, I've already paid for it (through my insurance)."

## HMOs

As insurance programs began to self-destruct because of overutilization and poor insurance judgments, a new concept began to evolve—that of the "health maintenance organization" (HMO), or as it has now become more generally known, "managed care." The original idea was not implausible. The HMO would focus on prevention of illness through comprehensive care and thereby largely dispense with control of quality and cost as intrinsic features. As it has turned out, however, the prevention of illness is much more under the control of patients than of healthcare professionals, so the expected cost savings have not been evident. Smoking, drinking, obesity, and indolence were seen to be among the most important precursors of illness, yet medical care, however managed, has been largely unsuccessful in altering them.

Worse still for the managed care concept, it began to become clear that perverse incentives governed care delivery. Planners and managers, operating out of the tradition of the business school and the ethics of the marketplace, had little incentive to develop systems of high durability. Their most important personal goals were those of high financial compensation which, in turn, made a strong positive cash flow imperative. This imperative produced its own logic of patient selection, namely to attract healthy subscribers using demographics and advertising techniques, to prevent the sick from signing with the plan, and to extrude current subscribers who become seriously ill. Once the logic was in place, HMOs became highly competitive with each other, encouraging, among other things their sicker members to leave the plan and go to competitors. High dropout rates and chaotic turnover followed. Further, deceiving patients about the quality of the care they were being provided became an important tool; for example, many physicians were forced to agree to "gag rules" which prevented them from providing patients with their best advice. Soon, managers' approval of the cost-effectiveness of a treatment became mandatory policy, and physicians who objected to managers' decisions could be extruded from the plan.[3]

The bottom line to the preceding points is that managed care insurance and indemnity insurance both have pitfalls that in the long run create an unacceptable instability in healthcare. The essential lesson in both cases is the failure to recognize that medical care is not a fungible commodity and that its delivery cannot ignore a moral basis. A mechanism—one might even say an admirable mechanism—designed to compensate for unexpected loss through risk sharing simply turns out to be inadequate to the task of covering costs for routine and expected events.

## The Free Market Solution

If price controls, government programs, and insurance in its many forms cannot produce high-quality care at reasonable costs, and if there is not substantial equality of access, then why not use the traditional American way of the free market? Although this is undoubtedly part of the healthcare solution as well as one of its necessary conditions, it is not in itself a sufficient condition. Individual freedom and responsibility is a deeply imprinted mental legacy for us, but there are other considerations as well. For example, although the welfare of children is fundamentally the responsibility of parents, the community has an interest and obligation to guarantee a child's welfare as well. It is simply not acceptable by our moral standards for a parent to decide that scarce dollars will be spent on beer rather than on a child's immunizations. Thus, as a society we insist that parents provide for the reasonable healthcare of their children. That is, we insist that individual choice be tempered with a prudent concern for the welfare of the society as a whole, for the welfare of the children of our society, for the welfare of those persons lacking in capacity to care for themselves, and that all citizens fulfill basic responsibilities consistent with the maintenance of public health. Contagious diseases must be treated, basic nutritional needs must be met, and water and air must be guarded to insure purity. All these necessary features of a healthcare system must flow from ethical considerations beyond a purely free market. We return to these points below.

## Technological Solution

For the past 300 years, Western civilization has counted the flowering of the scientific worldview and the development of technology as its crowning achievement. Wealth has been created and knowledge has been enhanced to a degree never before imagined. Progress is now taken for granted as part of the human legacy. Medicine in particular, and healthcare in general, have been among the most salient beneficiaries. The weekly announcement of new drugs and diagnostic/intervention procedures is a routine and expected feature of life.

How is it, then, that such strong opposition has arisen to technological development? That is, how has it come to be that the explosion of healthcare costs is largely attributed to technological progress? Implicit in this criticism is the assumption that there is some ideal level of technological advancement, and that we must not progress beyond it, lest we incur unacceptable expense. Healthcare planners often note the correlation between rising costs and the use of enhanced and superior new techniques. From this correlation, they erroneously assume causality. How can it be that technological enterprise and its consequent improvement of treatment somehow, in this unique case, make costs rise, while in literally every other example of technological advances, quality and availability are enhanced while costs decline?

Clearly, something is wrong here. It just doesn't seem plausible that healthcare is such a unique feature of human experience that we need special rules to defend us from rapacious technology and its explosive costs, while similar advancement in other field brings about higher quality, wider distribution, and lower cost. If improved technology and higher costs are correlated, and yet their causal connection is implausible, then there must be a confounding issue that needs to be identified. Some perverse force or forces must be raising costs and preventing scientific advancement from performing its usual role of wealth enhancement. What these perverse forces are is one of the major themes of this book. For now, let us say that they have to do with incentives buried in the system which divert efficient capital flow from central concerns toward essentially parasitic activities. To cite but one example, a number of perfectly legal companies work primarily to instruct hospitals and healthcare providers about how to maximally gouge Medicare by identifying and exploiting ambiguities in its payment rules.[4]

In their zeal to create a utopian system of free, perfect, and universally available healthcare, many planners have suggested that technology is the problem and must, somehow, be rolled back. Even the most cursory inquiry suggests that such a recommendation is fatuous. Which kinds of knowledge, and which applications of it, should be suppressed? Exactly which drugs and procedures should we eliminate? How far back should we go? Shall we begin again to apply leeches? Shall we resume bloodletting? Yes, these would be cheaper than modern antibiotics. But they wouldn't work, and that counts for something.

New technology may, indeed, cause increases in costs. Yet not all cost increases are bad. If productivity is enhanced to an even greater degree, then a good thing has happened. Said another way, there is no economic or moral equivalence between productivity-related costs and the mushrooming costs of new layers of non-productive administrators. Nevertheless, for now, we have to face the fact that high technology is not doing its usual good job for the healthcare enterprise. Although in our view any society would be foolish to argue for a moratorium on the discovery and application of new knowledge, until we identify better means of having technology work for us in this area—this is, until we reduce perverse incentives—each advance is potentially problematic. Technology is a necessary condition for the solution to our healthcare problems, yet it remains far from a sufficient condition.

## Return to Past Glory

The return to an imagined golden age of medical care has undeniable nostalgic appeal. Norman Rockwell once drew the pictures which many of us carry in our minds from childhood. A caring, avuncular physician sits at his rolltop desk, the dangling stethoscope a reassuring talisman to the child whose toy animal needs medical care. This was a world in which there were no bad outcomes and no illness that could not be cured. Somehow, the doctor would make it all turn out all right. No money ever changed hands. Of course, no one expected perfection. We knew that the human condition meant that people die, but that would be a long time away, and maybe someone would invent something. And certainly no one ever sued anyone else—that would be bad manners. Doctors still made house calls and brought cure sometimes, and hope and caring always. They carried pills in their black leather bags and gave them to you at no extra charge. Rarely, a prescription had to be filled at the drugstore, with its marble-topped soda fountain somehow reassuring us that the story would end well.

Clearly, this vision never existed. If it had, we would still expect more today. Greater knowledge brings with it greater expectation. We have similar fondness for the childhood memories of shopping at the corner grocery store, with its familiar, reassuring smells, its open pickle barrel, its aproned proprietor reaching to the top shelf with a long-handled clamp. Yet we also know that supermarkets have greater variety, lower unit cost, improved hygiene, easier accessibility, higher quality, faster service, and readily available parking.

Efficiencies and economies of scale make the return to the piece-work past of medical care just as problematic. Systems evolve. Sometimes they lose their way and require midcourse corrections. This is one of those times. There is a way to embrace the promise of modern scientific medicine with high quality, substantial equity, and costs controlled by self-correcting mechanisms. To find this way, we must look to what we now know of the behavior of people, individually and in groups.

## Myths of Quality Control

The science and art of quality control has been an important feature of industry for decades. More recently, healthcare services have recognized the importance of using systematic mechanisms for quality measurement and improvement. It is not, then, surprising that the methods found useful in industry have been grafted onto healthcare systems in a way that tends to assume some sort of equivalence. Whether this will prove to be an acceptable strategy for the long run remains to be seen, however. As we have noted, healthcare is not a fungible commodity, and so definitions of quality remain somewhat elusive. There are, nevertheless, some general principles of quality management that may be borrowed from other disciplines.

### Good versus Cheap versus Fast

Every engineer knows that products of his design will be evaluated from three points of view simultaneously. Customers want to know whether a device will perform according to promise, what its cost will be, and when it will be delivered. Thus every engineering design must consider trade-offs and compromises because it is not possible to maximize all three parameters simultaneously. The customer can have performance and low cost, but delivery time may be extended. We can offer rapid delivery of a quality product at an increased cost. Or we can produce a device quickly and cheaply but it won't work very well.[5]

Unfortunately, many healthcare planners are not satisfied with the three points model. Facts are often difficult to face, and contemplation of the limits of medical treatment often invites return to the reveries of our childhood—if we wish hard enough, we will be rewarded. Alas, it is not so. To seek the perfection of our childhood expectations is to abandon the practical compromises on which our well-being and freedom largely depend. In healthcare, as in politics, to seek perfection is to abandon the best possible solution at the time. The history of this century demonstrates to the most stubborn among us that utopian solutions invite catastrophe. Hasn't it been said that "Inside every perfection-seeking idealist is a totalitarian trying to emerge?"

Another cause of confusion in quality control is the lack of consensus on the limits of the quality. Two competing models exist to describe the task. Healthcare professionals most frequently see the problem as a matter of treatment of disease, while patients tend to view their distress in the larger context of illness. Disease is a matter of the scientific understanding of disordered biology, while the concept of illness considers the human impact of the pathologic process. Illness thus includes the family and the social context as well as expected changes over time. Both models in part are anchored in truth. There are forms of pathology that family and social context will not cure. And the treatment of disordered biology is likely to fail if the impact on loving relationships and working capacity is not considered.

Unfortunately, methods of quality assessment fail to address the fact that there are two models, each partially true. It is hard to measure quality in the scientific treatment of disease because diagnosis cannot always be precise, and conditions with the same label often vary greatly in severity. It is harder still to measure quality of life within the social and emotional impact of illness. For example, how many quality units is it worth to be able to walk? Does a thin smoker have better health than an obese non-smoker? Do serious treatable diseases count for more or less than milder chronic illnesses?

Does an empathic physician deserve more or fewer quality points than a brusque but highly skilled surgeon? Can all the healthcare professions be measured on the same scale? Does a major university hospital a hundred miles away have a higher operational utility than a local community hospital? These questions serve as examples of the practical difficulties inherent in any fair and useful measurement of total quality.

Just as there is a lack of consensus on the definition of quality, there is also confusion on means of correction and improvement. Should there be more or less intervention and control by government? Should there be more physicians or fewer? Should they have more or less education and training? Does the law of supply and demand apply to physicians?[6] Does the quality of a physician's skill vary with the number of them? Does this matter? Are all physicians equally skilled, or at least sufficiently skilled? Is insurance the preferred mode of payment, or should there be more direct responsibility for the costs by having patients pay directly? Should government pay for everything? If so, should it be by means of social security or general revenue? And what about confidentiality? Is it critically necessary, or only desirable, or unimportant? Is the Joint Commission on Accreditation of Healthcare Organizations (JCAHO) a necessary guarantor of quality? Is it sufficient? Should it have competitors for quality assurance, or should it be a monopoly?

There are even more central questions for which we have no clear answers. Should everyone receive the same standard of care, regardless of financial considerations? If you believe that the answer to this question is yes, then are you prepared to say that those of more substantial means should be forbidden from making private contracts with providers who operate outside a government or insurance-based plan?[7] Moreover, how might this be enforced? And is this idea consistent with the general American consensus that people should be able to spend their money as they please? On the other hand, if you believe that it is acceptable to have more than one standard of care, then where should lines of quality be drawn? Should all be entitled to emergency care but not to routine or elective care? How do we define an emergency? How should we apply this policy to the needs of children? How about the elderly and the mentally impaired? Are some lives worth more than others? Who decides?

## One Attempt at Quality Control—The Deming Method

Many in the world of commerce and industry are familiar with the work of W. Edwards Deming, a celebrated management consultant whose fame has spread since his methods were embraced by Japanese corporations during their postwar recovery. The Deming method appears highly compatible with the virtues commonly associated with the Japanese style—enthusiastic group solidarity and cooperation. One of the central assumptions of the method is that quality may be defined as the progressive reduction of variance. In other words, a production run that has units which vary within a narrow range has an inherently higher quality than one in which the range is wider. Whatever innovations in quality enhancement may occur will consist of new methods of variance reduction and promotion of uniformity of the product. These new methods are expected to come from committees, which arrive at them in a democratic spirit and a nonhierarchical setting.

The quality of many products from Japan is eloquent testimony to the effectiveness of this method. Electronic components and automobiles do indeed appear to increase in quality and availability while enjoying stable or decreasing price. But is this method equally valid for other types of production? Can it be a universal standard that insures the continued enhancement of quality in all areas of human achievement? Many seem to think so. Corporate offices and government bureaus at every level have embraced this fad with wide-eyed enthusiasm. An industry has emerged which consists of trainers who claim that they are skilled in the method. Yet any skepticism is ignored or scornfully turned aside. When skepticism does rear its ugly head, the usual argument runs along the lines of "well, look, the boss has decided to do this, and everyone is expected to cooperate." The tyranny of the group mind takes hold, even though ironically the whole idea began with the presumption of free inquiry at every level of the organization.

Certainly the reduction of variance is an important aspect of quality for lots of things, such as the production of ball bearings—although it is important that they be of the right size as well as uniform size. To subject a more complex production process to the reduction of variance approach is to invite some amusing paradoxes. For example, consider the case of a master painter or sculptor who is expected to define the quality of his work in terms of its uniformity. The same point applies to healthcare providers; not to consider individual variation both as a feature of patients and of treatments is to assure a reduction in quality. In effect, making the case for variance reduction becomes less important to the degree that production involves complex products or services—especially those products or services that must consider judgments or values.

It seems reasonable to conclude that the Deming method and those like it, at least in their currently practiced American form, have limited value for quality enhancement for the changing healthcare environment. Medical care may not rise to the creative standards of the great masters, but neither is it analogous to a box of ball bearings. Not yet, anyway. Where freedom, judgment, and progress are important, we will have to look elsewhere to understand what quality might mean and how it might be pursued. Perhaps JCAHO is the answer.

## The Joint Commission on Accreditation and Healthcare Organizations (JCAHO)

This independent and nonprofit organization performs assessments of quality of care on a voluntary basis for hospitals and other institutional providers. Originally formed as a consortium by the American Medical Association, the American Colleges of Medicine and Surgery, and the American Hospital Association, it has for decades provided consultative surveys on issues of quality. At first, JCAHO accreditation was considered an elective, although highly desirable, marker of excellence. As funding by insurance companies and government programs has assumed a dominant position in healthcare, the JCAHO seal of approval has become essential. Although the surveys remain formally voluntary, no provider can now survive without successful completion of this periodic rite of passage, since virtually all reimbursement is contingent upon accreditation. The cost of these triennial surveys is borne by the hospitals. The surveys are wide-ranging and comprehensive in their scope, and successful passage requires rigorous vigilance to compliance with a vast compendium of detailed regulations. Thus JCAHO provides a uniform standard of care for a very diverse group of healthcare providers.

Although much good work is accomplished by these efforts, we cannot leave the problem of quality assurance to this mechanism. But why? The answer is not difficult. Over time JCAHO has become an autonomous bureaucracy which sees itself as having the final word on just what quality is. There is no competition from other accrediting bodies, and thus no effective feedback to insure that the regulations remain practical, pertinent, and cost-effective. JCAHO therefore has very substantial authority over a hospital's resource allocation. This leaves the hospital with the responsibility for maintaining quality and financial stability, while JCAHO has de facto authority but no responsibility, and thus it is not cost-sensitive. If the survey recommends a particular quality measure, then the hospital must comply with it, regardless of cost. Over time, resource allocation is skewed toward those measures of quality currently in vogue in the higher councils of JCAHO, which may not always be congruent with the best state-of-the-art practice. Standardization comes at the price of procrustean regulation, from which the provider has no capacity for substantive appeal. The quality assessment effort would be shaped toward more effective compromises if JCAHO had a competitor commission with parallel authority to confer accreditation, and thus reimbursement, from third-party payers.

As it now stands, JCAHO sets standards that many see as arbitrary. It remains the sole judge of acceptable compliance with standards. If the hospital fails to be accredited, it must correct the purported quality deficiency or go out of business. JCAHO will help with consultation, for a fee. It will also decide how often, and how comprehensive, the surveys will be. Thus,

JCAHO decides how often and how much the hospital will pay them, and there is no effective appeal. Some cynics have suggested a structural resemblance to a protection racket.

## Alternative Therapies

If mainstream medicine is difficult to evaluate for quality, the wonderland of "alternative therapies" remains impervious to the most rigorous attempts at investigation. Having at last lifted itself out of the mysticism of the past, scientific medicine seemed invulnerable to criticism of its underlying principles of observation and logic. Yet over the past quarter century the consensus that scientific thinking is the best way to discover truth was itself undermined. Folkways have always been important in matters such as home remedies, and superstition has been a frequent companion. Until recently, the government, the foundations, the universities, and private enterprise could be expected to know that science is better than magic for solving problems. Nevertheless, in recent years this broad consensus of educated people has broken down. One of us has had the experience, while chairman of a department of a major teaching hospital, of being presented with a crystal with purported therapeutic value—not by a patient, but by another faculty member. It was not easy to fight back a wave of despair. Alternative medical systems—that is, those that eschew logical analysis—have enjoyed a resurgence that is as breathtaking as it is hard to explain.[8]

The variety of these purported therapies is extensive. New and old forms of mumbo jumbo happily co-exist. Homeopathy and chiropractic, herbal medicine and therapeutic touch, psychic healing and crystal power, acupuncture and reflexology, all enjoy a respectability that emerges from some deep wellspring of wishful thinking that is part of the human condition. The Enlightenment was supposed to have changed all that, at least among the educated and the serious-minded. Yet, in many ways, we seem to be marching back into the bad old days when truth was whatever suited the strongest or the most unscrupulous. How can this be? Why would the educated, the influential, the strong, all allow themselves to be so beguiled? As always, when a phenomenon of such powerful foolishness occurs, one must look for incentives that drive the system away from clarity and toward primitive prelogical ideas.[9]

Some of these incentives are easy to identify. For example, pharmacies are tempted to sell water in small glass vials. They claim them as homeopathic medicines because there is an enormously greater profit margin than that which comes from selling real drugs whose retail price has been driven below cost by managed care contracting schemes. The rationale is, of course, that this is only giving the people what they want. But traditionally the people have been led to expect that professionals would not mislead them. When medical care is dispensed by a few large corporations, then it is quickly recognized by the profit-maximizers that alternative means of care, although ineffective, are cheaper, at least in the short run—and for the corporation, the short run is all that counts. After all, they can delude themselves into thinking that meeting people's wants is somehow equivalent to treatment. Of course, water in small glass vials is not giving the people what they want. People want medical treatments that work.

## Tort Law and Malpractice Lawsuits

One of the articles of faith of the American Trial Lawyers Association is that the practice of aggressive prosecution of civil torts promotes improved quality of professional practice. Trial lawyers traditionally assert that were it not for their vigilant attention all manner of mistakes would go unnoticed, and thus quality of service in medical and other matters would be impaired. This is, to say the least, an unproved hypothesis. What we do know is that there is a lot of malpractice that goes undetected, while there is a lot of good practice that is vilified by frivolous lawsuits because of an unfortunate outcome. Quality control by tort litigation is a very blunt instrument indeed. Once again we are faced with the concept that truth is whatever we want it to be—that is, that fault exists if something bad happens, and the fault resides in the person with the most money. We all know in our hearts that this is a meretricious concept, serving neither truth nor justice. That it remains a routine practice illustrates the viscosity of the political process and the tenacity of the self-interest of the trial lawyers.

## Root Causes of Healthcare Myths

As we examine the myths and confusions which have become part of the healthcare environment, two underlying themes appear. The first is that we have apparently relaxed our insistence that the scientific mode of thought is preferable to that of authority, faith, and magic for solving the kinds of problems that emerge. The causes of this phenomenon are beyond the scope of this book, but it must be said that we have no hope of developing a more rational system until we remember that reason is our indispensable ally. In practical terms, we need to reduce the influence of politicians on healthcare decisions, because the modern politician seems determined to tell us what we want to hear. Because the character of politicians is unlikely to exceed that of the electorate, we can only hope for a rediscovered ethos of individual responsibility.

The other theme at the root of our difficulty is the inherent conflict between our twin imperatives of seeking freedom and seeking equality. Though both ideals are worthy of pursuit, to insist on simultaneous perfection in each for healthcare is just not going to work. We need to develop a consensus for compromise.

## CONCLUDING COMMENTS

Given the key points in this chapter, what is to be done? A system that would have a plausible chance of major improvement would be decentralized, locally managed, and would allow for competition. Practitioners would be responsible for quality management. Governance would be congruent with what is now known of group behavior. Patients would have incentive to be sensitive to costs. They would insist on getting what they pay for, and be willing to pay for what they get.[10]

## NOTES

1. Government has in some ways departed from the role of honest broker and has become an interest group in its own right. See, for example, B. Fagin, *Skeptical Inquirer*, May–June 1997. In this short article he discusses the necessity for a data-driven and fact-based approach to political questions, drawing on the public-choice theory of Nobelist James Buchanan.

2. Insurance has a tendency to obscure the purpose of the therapeutic encounter. In the *Wall Street Journal*, 12 September 1997, N. Jeffries identifies the jungle of complexity that insurance claims have created.

3. There is an assumption implicit in the managed care concept that medical care can be reduced to economic and business decisions. See an editorial by R. Goldberg of George Washington University in the *Wall Street Journal*, 18 June 1997.

4. L. Lagnado details how consultants have squeezed the Medicare system in the *Wall Street Journal*, 10 February 1998.

5. In a two-part health policy report, T. Bodenheimer details some of the lessons from the Oregon Health Plan and its challenges dealing with the logical constraints on cost, access, and quality. See the *New England Journal of Medicine*, 28 August and 4 September 1997.

6. Politicians never tire of trying to repeal the laws of supply and demand. In the *New York Times*, 25 August 1997, W. Leary describes how some of America's premier teaching hospitals are being paid by government to reduce the supply of medical specialists.

7. It is hard to find a more clear example of the idea that the government seems to believe that it owns our bodies. In the *Wall Street Journal*, 22 August 1997, the editors call attention to newly advanced Medicare policy which would effectively deny to those over age 65 the right to make private contracts with physicians for care.

8. It must also be kept in mind that the "alternative" treatments have been part of folklore since before the beginning of history. R. Henig in *Civilization*, April/May 1997, discusses medicine's "New Age" therapies, pointing out that evaluation of effectiveness is the critical challenge. But this is just what alternative practitioners can't or won't do, since they eschew the scientific method.

9. In the *Skeptical Inquirer*, September–October 1997, B. Beyerstein discusses the methodological problems in the evaluation of alternative therapies.

10. Medical Savings Accounts, properly designed and enabled by appropriate legislation, would appear to avoid many of the pitfalls discussed in this chapter. Needless to say, the concept is vigorously opposed by special interests, including some elements of government. See G. Scandlen, *Wall Street Journal*, 15 September 1997.

*Chapter 4*

# The Current State of US Healthcare

You ask how I spend my time and what satisfaction I receive from my work. . . . Are you sure you want the answers? First of all, time is always an issue. . . . Half of my working day [12 hours per day, 5 days per week, and 6 hours on Saturday] is spent trying to maintain quality. . . . That usually means saying the same thing time and again to staff that have other things on their mind. . . . It's not so difficult to care for the elderly if you follow a few rules. . . . But the staff has other concerns, like whether they will get their break, which among them is not carrying his or her load, and the usual gossip items. . . . At times I want to yell, to tell them if they would simply do their work correctly they would have plenty of time for other things. . . . Then there is the third of my day that I spend arguing with project administrators, whose only reason for existence seems to be to say no to any suggestion that the project put quality of care at the top of its priority list—it's depressing. . . . With the time that is left, I do paper work, much of which I end up taking home because there is simply too much to do. . . . I won't be in this job long—I'm already burned out.

> Interview with a 34-year-old physician, first in his class in
> college and medical school, an associate professor at one of
> American's premier medical schools, and director of a group
> of physicians and caretakers responsible for the medical care of
> several thousand elderly patients in residential living projects

## INTRODUCTION

No complex system will be perfect. The US healthcare system—"systems" is a more accurate term—is no exception. Yet there are degrees of perfection, and recognizing what works and what does not work in any system is a prerequisite to identifying where change is necessary. Evaluating our healthcare system will not be easy. Many of the supposed "facts" offered by politicians, healthcare payers, healthcare providers, and patient/disease interest groups do little more than confuse and obscure our most fundamental healthcare problems. Where then does one start? First, by looking at the better points of healthcare today.

## HEALTHCARE—THE GOOD POINTS

Perhaps the least controversial feature of modern medicine is its technical side. Despite some calls for a moratorium on technology, the diagnostic and investigative capacities of PET and MRI, the precise anatomical and chemical analysis of tissues, the characterizing of genes and their effects, the creative modeling of computers, and the ever-increasing specificity of drugs are but a few examples of technology's contribution to today's medicine.[1] One may question some of the paths (e.g., drug experimentation on animals) by which these contributions have made their way to the forefront of medicine, yet from almost any perspective they represent impressive technological accomplishments. Further accomplishments can be expected in the future.

Improvements in precision of clinical diagnosis and treatment have a similar history. Compared to even a decade ago, clinicians are better able to characterize and identify many diseases and disorders, to predict accurately their clinical course, and to intervene in ways that are beneficial to patients. The updating and dissemination of knowledge also gets a strong positive review. Journals, books, the Internet, special TV channels, the Library of Congress, and required continuing medical education are excellent sources and venues for the rapid dissemination of information about new clinical and research findings.

These good points are not matters of happenstance. Thousands of hours go into perfecting each technical advance, improving and validating new diagnoses, testing and comparing the efficacy of different treatments, and collating, interpreting, and disseminating information. The decline in deaths among persons with AIDS is one outcome of such efforts.[2] Likewise, each day thousands of doctor–patient encounters take place. The majority of these encounters accomplish their healthcare goals, indicating that there is both purpose and order in much of our healthcare system.

Also on the positive side, many of the best minds in the country continue to enter healthcare fields. Far more people apply to medical school than are accepted. US medical training is still among the world's best, and ethical standards, though eroding, are still important to a percentage of providers and aspiring clinicians.

Added together, these points could be taken as signs that our healthcare system is better than its critics contend. The negative press that healthcare often receives may reflect a journalistic bias in which reporters as well as critics are unrealistic about the level of healthcare perfection achievable in a country of 260 million people. Possibly! Yet, remain skeptical. There is simply too much evidence suggesting otherwise. Despite its many good points, and despite the work of thousands of individuals trying to achieve quality medical care, our healthcare system is far from what it could or should be. Parts of the system work at cross-purposes and lack direction. Fraud and excessive profit-taking exists. Quality of care differs significantly from location to location. There are indefensible delays and denials of treatment. For many of these problems, there are no indications that change is in the wind.[3]

## HEALTHCARE—THE BAD POINTS

Historically, many of the features of today's healthcare can be traced to the years following World War II and the emergence of perverse incentives which have corrupted people and systems.

Practical factors were in part responsible for bringing these incentives into play. The effects of the educational years lost in World War II and the cost of medical education provide convenient examples. By the time many aspiring doctors had spent several years in the armed forces, paid for college, medical school, and postdoctoral training in a medical specialty (e.g., surgery, internal medicine), their financial debts were well into six figures. There was a need to repay their loans and to have money to start and raise families. That young doctors, many of whom had completed 24 years of education, wanted for the first time in their adult lives to be on a solid financial footing is not surprising. Nor is it surprising that many were attracted to those areas of medicine that paid well or promised to do so. Through the 1950s and 1960s, slowly, yet perceptibly, the costs for their services increased. Physicians charged more for their services. For the first time in the history of American medicine the average clinician could become wealthy and not just earn a respectable income. As the price of medicine rose, the American Medical Association (AMA) and the associations representing medical specialties (e.g., surgery, radiology, anesthesiology) remained silent.

Some doctors spotted these trends early on and tried to convince their colleagues that undesirable consequences would follow. Their concerns had little effect. Unnecessary medical consultations and surgical procedures continued and the dollars followed. Critics from outside of healthcare began to raise their voices. Something was morally wrong with doctors becoming wealthy as the expense of others' suffering. This criticism was not new; it had been leveled against morticians for centuries. By 1970, drug companies would begin to hear their share of such criticism. Nor could rising costs of providers' services be tolerated indefinitely. The 1980s would bring major changes, as insurance companies, HMOs, and the federal and state governments with Medicare and Medicaid began implementing price controls for physicians' services.

The cost of providers' services was only one issue, however. What bothered critics as much as the rising costs of treatment was the fact that medicine was substituting economic rationalizations for traditional medical ethics. "Where art thou Hippocrates?" one critic asked. To this and other questions, medicine stood its ground. It was a seller's market from the 1950s through the 1970s. The medical community countered with arguments that its members were financially deserving and immune from normal ethical standards. One author of the time summed up the critics views in the following way, "The divorce between medicine and morality has been defended on the ground that medical categories, unlike those of law and religion, rest on scientific foundations exempt from moral evaluation".[4] The frequently heard term "conflict of interest" is about this very point.

Government and private foundation funding introduced its own set of perverse incentives. The post–World War II era saw a major infusion of such funding into medical research, and many of the technical accomplishments discussed thus far had their birth during the period between 1950 and 1980. It is to these decades that the origins of many impressive biological findings can be traced, with the genetic and physiological causes of diseases being perhaps the most impressive.

Other sides to the funding story existed. For example, academics receiving extramural funds (grants and contracts from sources outside the institution in which they worked) could increase their salaries. In turn, their university appointments were often accelerated. Funds meant power, influence, and control, and, in some instances, research dynasties emerged. Universities and research institutes quickly picked up on the idea that extramural funding could provide a welcome source of income ("overhead costs") that could be used for a variety of purposes other than research. Because government funding units and private foundations often paid (and still pay) significant overhead costs—at times equal to the amount of money allocated for research—universities and research institutes found themselves competing as much for the overhead dollars as for the privilege of conducting research. Successful competition often required hiring a host of young investigators as well as the occasional senior researcher (and supporting personnel) who had already established worth in attracting funds. Medical investigators were on the move.

Every type of funding has its day; government and private funding would not turn out to be exceptions. Funding for medical research was at its height in the mid-1970s. By the 1980s, it was leveling off. Undaunted by the limitation of funds, more and more researchers and institutions jumped into the funding arena to compete for their slice of the shrinking resource pie. The outcomes of these events—more investigators and institutions competing for a fixed amount of research money—could have been predicted had anyone taken the time to do a few simple calculations. Universities and research institutions began downsizing; academic unemployment began to rise. With these changes, there appeared a new academic breed, the "elite unsupported," composed of investigators, once well-funded, but no longer attractive targets for the deep pockets of funding brokers.

Physicians' salaries and funding details aside, from the end of World War II through the mid-1980s, healthcare was the high road for many young Americans. More and more students applied to medical, nursing, and graduate schools. For medicine, the number of applicants far exceeded the opportunities for admission. Medical schools could count on full classes and, to a large degree, pick and choose the applicants they wished to train. Like funding, the greater the total number of applicants to medical schools, the greater the competition for admission and the greater the number of applicants rejected—medical schools have their own enrollment limits. With the popularity of medical education increasing, medical school admission committees began to feel the strain of processing thousands of applications. Enter the MCAT. The Medical College Admissions Test (MCAT) consists of a series of moderately difficult questions, puzzles, and comprehension assessments. First developed during the 1950s, this test would become a prominent part of screening candidates for medical school. The personal interview, on the other hand, became less important.

In principle, there is probably more good than bad about having a test for prospective medical students. Tests serve to screen out those students who are unable to master the academic material required of today's healthcare providers. Tests also help to identify the exceptional student. A high score on the MCAT, when combined with an A average from college, not only promises admission to medical school, but it also means that a student has a high probability of completing his or her medical training. Lower MCAT scores and/or college grades reduce one's opportunities for admission and graduation accordingly. If nothing else, the MCAT can be defended as having leveled the playing field for medical school admission.

Yet answering questions and puzzles and scoring well on comprehension assessments are not all there is to being a quality healthcare provider. In the case of the MCAT, it became too easy for members of medical school admissions committees to overvalue "the test" and to admit applicants primarily on the basis of their college grades and MCAT scores.

The troublesome side of reducing medical school admission to a set of numbers (college grades and test scores) is simply this: it downgrades the value of an applicant's humanity and motivation to cure the ill, while it upgrades the value of cognitive dexterity and the ability to memorize. By "humanity" we mean that providers take the time to understand patients, that they take the time to communicate clearly to patients the reasons for their suffering, and that they design medical interventions in ways that patients are likely to accept and follow. Humanity also means that providers are available to reconfigure treatments that do not work as originally planned (somewhere between 40–60%) And humanity means that providers are able to find personal rewards in carrying out these activities.

Few of medicine's detractors would argue that cognitive dexterity and the ability to memorize are unimportant attributes for clinicians. Likewise, many of those who support the MCAT as an admission-screening tool do not claim that cognitive attributes necessarily translate into clinical humanity. All well and good. But then, what does one do with the fact that approximately half of the success of the average medical intervention hinges on human factors. Patients need to feel that their doctors are truthful, empathetic, and inclined to do what is necessary to improve their health.

Our purpose in discussing the MCAT is not to have the test eliminated. Rather, it is to call attention to an important change in medicine, namely the increasing dependence on numbers in preference to other types of attribute assessments in medical decision making. No matter where one looks, from medical school admissions, to the overhead for funding applications, to the number of patients treated per day by an HMO provider, numbers are what counts. If numbers are all there is to healthcare, the healthcare dilemma should be easy to solve—most of us can add and subtract. But there must be something more to healthcare than numbers.

## HEALTHCARE STATISTICS

If one tries to get a reading on healthcare today, one immediately confronts a litany of success and horror stories embedded in mounds of statistics.[5] Many believe that if a percentage or a probability can be assigned to an act, an idea, a symptom, or a treatment, understanding will increase and interventions will be more effective. When numbers are offered as proxies for real events, some numbers are more meaningful and informative than others are. For example, it makes sense to talk in terms of numbers when dealing with the percentage of school children who have not been immunized, the number of new AIDS cases during the previous year, and the number of individuals over 65 who suffer from dementia. Conversely, it makes little sense to apply numbers to quality of care assessments, to patients' willingness to cooperate with providers, or to the emotional impact of disease on family members.

Given these words of caution, take a quick look at a few of the statistics dealing with US healthcare. Some have weathered scrutiny; some will change. Many hint at the kinds of problems that any aspiring healthcare system needs to address.

- While declining, infant morality rates still remain high in the United States, somewhere around 7 per 1,000 live births.

- Approximately 2 million unnecessary operations are performed each year in the United States, and a percentage of these operations result in patient deaths.[6]
- Significant racial/ethnic differences exist in the percentage of children who are immunized, the percentage of adults who develop diseases (e.g., hypertension, heart disease), and in dental care.
- Thirty-five million Americans lack some type of health insurance.[7]
- Among low-, medium-, and high-income groups, significant differences occur in the prevalence and seriousness of chronic health conditions.
- More than twice as many people with schizophrenia and manic-depressive psychosis live in public shelters or on the streets than in mental hospitals.
- Most community mental health centers have been abysmal failures.
- Although the number of persons with private health insurance has leveled off, insurance company and HMO premiums for healthcare continue to increase, while the healthcare services they provide (diagnosis and treatment) have either not improved or have declined.[8]
- Over 5% of individuals 75–84 years of age are in nursing homes, and over 20% of persons 85 years and older are in nursing homes.
- The cost of prescription drugs consistently outpaces inflation, and this causes increases in the overall costs of medical care. Drug prices for the same or comparable drugs in the United States exceed those of Western Europe by a factor of three to one. Return on stockholder equity among drug companies is nearly twice that of the average return for *Fortune* 500 companies.
- The percentage of average family income spent on healthcare was 9% in 1980, 11.7% in 1991, and is projected at 16.4% for the year 2000. Anticipated HMO cost increases in the next few years range from 10% to 15%.
- Selected contagious diseases such as tuberculosis and genital herpes continue to increase in number, while other diseases such as AIDS and some forms of heart disease are on the decline.
- Medications are responsible for approximately 100,000 deaths per year.
- Medicare's austerity leads to more elderly joining frugal HMOs.[9]
- Although estimates vary, studies repeatedly suggest that, at a minimum, 15% of medical care is suboptimal.

No matter what slant one gives to these statistics, it is difficult to argue that any one of them can be taken as an indication that our healthcare system is operating optimally. Some chronicle the consequences of past events. This is the case, for example, with community mental health centers and the fact that currently a significant number of mentally ill persons are homeless and untreated. While the sentiments responsible for this situation may have been well intended, perhaps 60% of the mentally ill persons who today wander the streets can be viewed as victims of the enthusiasm and persistence of misinformed citizen groups. "Free mental patients from the chains of the mental hospital" was a rallying cry for such groups. Legislative naivete concerning the seriousness of many forms of mental illness was profound. In other instances, statistics reflect quality of care issues, auditing practices, healthcare costs, government legislation and rule making, malpractice concerns, and fraud.

## QUALITY OF CARE

Statements about quality of care require close scrutiny. For example, patients are often uncertain about how to assess quality. Thus, their responses to surveys soliciting their views concerning the care they receive are likely to reflect a mixture of feelings and facts. Reports from healthcare providers raise yet other issues. Providers engaging in low-quality care are not likely to inform the public of their practices. Thus, their facts and figures are usually laced with deceptive information. On the other hand, those providers who practice quality medicine often inflate their successes and minimize their failures. Still, the finding that approximately 15% of healthcare is suboptimal certainly suggests that there is significant room for improvement.

Quality care requires time. Quality care is relevant to the disease or disorder from which a patient suffers. It is provided in a supportive context, and (except in emergencies) by known providers. Timeliness is important because not all medical problems are equally critical. Relevance is important because medical care that misses the mark can be dangerous to patients. A supportive environment is important because it reduces the fear and uncertainty that patients experience at moments when they are seeking medical care. Reducing uncertainty also significantly improves treatment outcome. And for patients to know healthcare providers is important because familiarity between patient and provider correlates with diagnostic accuracy and treatment effectiveness.[10]

Is quality of care a desired goal of literally everyone in and out of the healthcare system? The answer is yes—even the greediest medical entrepreneurs have no objection to quality medicine. Because quality of care is so universally desirable, its proponents, like the proponents of universal government-managed healthcare, are often bedfellows. Those who clamor for improved quality of care view themselves as saints while those who argue that quality can not be mandated or that new systems are required if quality is to be improved are either ignored, scorned, or both.

Both the saints and their detractors have their points. In theory, a government by the people and for the people should be able to provide a satisfactory healthcare system if the citizens want it badly enough. After all, Sweden, Canada, and Great Britain have somehow managed to develop satisfactory, although not always high-quality, healthcare systems. Yet theory is one thing, reality another. A fact of US life is that a similar solution is unlikely in the United States. There is simply too great a diversity of opinion, too much money and power at stake, and too many well-financed interest groups to lead to a national consensus, to nudge our healthcare system in novel directions, or to elevate it to acceptable levels of quality. When it comes to government-managed healthcare in the United States, it is wise to be realistic. Past history strongly suggests that this idea would be a very poor solution. If the postal or welfare services are examples, the US government has yet to prove that it can manage large service organizations efficiently and simultaneously maintain quality. Some other solution needs to be found.

Unfortunately, real causes of low-quality healthcare exist, some of which have their origins among providers. A poor medical education, the failure to remain aware of new medical information, indifference to patients' illnesses, and valuing the dollar more than providing a quality product are a few of the causes. Another is medical decision making. This means making judgments about which procedures should and could be used in diagnosing and treating diseases and disorders. Increasingly, medical judgments are out of the hands of clinicians and in the hands of government, insurance companies, and HMO administrators. Yet, only a handful of administrators are experienced in the delivery of care.[11] More important, there is literally no monitoring of their decision-making practices except as such practices influence cash flow. This provides an incentive for deceptive practices.[12]

## AUDITING PRACTICES

Yet another and somewhat paradoxical cause of compromised quality can be found in much of the behavior of oversight, audit, and quality control committees such as the Joint Commission on Accreditation of Healthcare Organizations (JCAHO), Medicare, the Occupational Safety and Health Administration (OSHA), and professional groups. On first pass, auditing practices seem to be a good idea and, as noted earlier, these groups have their place—things need to be reviewed! A closer look raises some questions, however, the most important of which deals with "criteria conflation" (in which each investigative body has its own special requirements and investigative criteria). For example, Medicare and Medicaid auditors are primarily concerned with whether the government is being cheated financially.[13] JCAHO reviewers are primarily concerned with whether medical records are in order, if employees have memorized their institution's motto, and if committee minutes are complete. OSHA is primarily concerned that the proper applications have been filed. In effect, there are too many regulators for too many diverse and competing groups! And regulators have little incentive to be guided by practical considerations.

If, on average, audits by JCAHO, Medicare, and so forth took only a few minutes a week, one could hardly object. Yet far too often even the most ethical and honest healthcare providers find themselves spending up to a half day a week addressing audit and review issues—and these demands increase daily. This is time lost to hands-on healthcare delivery, reeducation, and improving technical skills; it is costly in dollars because money has to be made elsewhere. Furthermore, audit and oversight committees invariably find it necessary to make recommendations or demands for changes; how else can they demonstrate that they are doing their job? Given that we have a far from perfect healthcare system, such recommendations are easy to develop. Yet recommendations are frequently made without any evidence that they are superior to procedures that are in place—like fashions, medicine is also subject to fads. Furthermore, poor recommendations are often accompanied by threats of years of probation, followed by loss of academic, hospital, or state licensing accreditation—each of which translate into the loss of cash and credibility.

## HEALTHCARE BY THE NUMBERS

If we allow that the audit and oversight groups were not invented to compromise the quality of healthcare (despite the fact that they often do so), it is another matter when we look at the ways that HMOs, insurance companies, and government agencies often think and act, bringing unfortunate consequences for quality healthcare.[14] Diseases and optimal treatment are far more complex than usually imagined. Moreover, much of this thinking reveals a surprising level of misunderstanding about the nuts and bolts of diagnosis and treatment. Much of this misunderstanding reflects the arrogance of the uninformed, particularly the assumption that various medical decisions can be assigned to the same category and manipulated from a cost perspective. The principle fallacy in such thinking is the assumption that it is possible to a achieve high degree of sameness and predictability in characterizing (1) patients (e.g., diagnosis), (2) patient flow (e.g., how patients move through systems), and (3) interventions (how patients are treated). Such thinking disregards the degree to which diseases, disorders, and humans differ. Trying to put people in neat little boxes is a waste of time if individual differences are at least half of what healthcare is about. This advent of diagnosis-cost-box thinking is a major contributor to the public's increasing interest in alternative forms of care, despite the fact that such care is unregulated, not tested for effectiveness, usually worthless, and only in rare instances reimbursed by insurance.

Clearly, attempts to categorize diseases and disorders in ways that suit the tastes of auditors, administrators, statisticians, and healthcare payers amount to little more than trying to conduct healthcare by assembly line. In principle, such attempts mirror the MCAT story. Such exercises simply ignore certain facts. Nature is complex; categories neither account for nor eliminate nature's complexity; no two patients or diseases are alike. Many diseases or disorders that are given the same diagnosis have different causes, and the same cause may result in very different signs and symptoms between two individuals. Pretending that nature is fathomable by using numbers invites misunderstanding, leads to erroneous statistics, supports suboptimal medical decisions, and assures that quality healthcare will not be achieved.

## HEALTHCARE COSTS

The cost of care is another major problem. HMOs and insurance companies can be more accurately characterized as resource-grabbing businesses rather than serious and purposeful healthcare organizations. They compete for clients, for cash, and for the control of providers, hospitals, and clinics. The organizations that have survived are highly competitive and at times ruthless. Those that have not survived, or will not, have often suffered from being too greedy.[15,16]

With increasing competition, the resource for which for-profit HMOs compete—cash—has become harder to come by. In turn, a standard formula is applied: decrease hospital admissions and reduce provider staffs. Once applied, the number of suboptimal medical evaluations increases, treatment options are restricted, and patients wait longer for services. In some instances, patient care is devastated. Study after study is consistent with this interpretation. For example, 42% of Californians with medical insurance, nearly all of whom are in managed care plans, had problems with their healthcare providers during 1996, including *thousands* who reported denials of treatment or delays in receiving treatment.[17] Unlike patient surveys dealing with quality of care, surveys dealing with denials of treatment or treatment delays are likely to be accurate.

Or take the case of mental illness. Managed care systems not only limit the amount of care they will provide, but hospital admissions of persons with mental illnesses are strictly limited to those who are imminently suicidal, homicidal, or unable to provide for their basic needs. Similar problems affect persons with chronic diseases (e.g., kidney disease) or specific genetic profiles, who also are frequently denied coverage. Such denials amount to arbitrary healthcare ostracism, similar to the treatment of persons with leprosy a century ago. Moreover they often end up costing more healthcare dollars and consuming more healthcare time than if they were treated. This is certainly the case with many mental illnesses that can be relatively inexpensively managed in terms of costs of drugs and provider time.

Economically, HMOs have turned out to be unstable organizations, a point suggested by their intense and often deceptive competition for clients, their frequent mergers, their revolving door policies regarding high-cost patients, their frequent rule changes, and their frequent denial of reasonable care. Organizational instability eventually leads to what some authors have termed "the organizational death cycle," a condition that develops when the inflow of resources from outside is insufficient to keep the organization running.[18]

**Figure 4.1**
**Increases in Medicaid and Medicare Costs between 1990 and 1998**

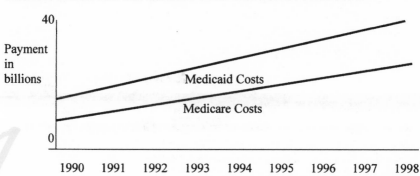

Much the same may be said about insurance companies. By their nature, they are actuarial in their thinking. They want to exclude those clients for whom the costs of healthcare delivery are likely to exceed the premiums clients pay. This is the basis of the above-mentioned revolving door policy: healthy patients are allowed to enter and costly patients are ushered out.

Given the preceding points, why then are senior citizens, in contrast to younger individuals, continuing to rush to join managed care programs that will accept Medicare payments? Part of the answer is that many HMOs as well as bogus advocacy groups have actively promoted this relationship because it provides them with a source of income. In effect, they are gambling on the fact that they can charge Medicare for the costs of the services they provide and still make a profit. But does the influx of senior citizens mean that they have identified sources of better quality care? We doubt it. More likely, the rush is better understood as the only operational choice open to many elderly.

The costs of governmental reimbursement for healthcare have also risen. Figure 4.1[19] shows the Medicare and Medicaid costs between 1990 and the present as well as the projected costs for 1998. Note that the costs have more than doubled between 1990 and 1997, and they are slated to increase once again in 1998.

What are the sources of these costs? Some have been mentioned. Others need to be identified. There are, first of all, legitimate costs. Healthcare takes time and requires the use of multiple personnel with different skills. For example, the use of PET and MRI equipment is far more expensive than taking an x ray and requires the use of highly trained technicians. Machines require frequent servicing. Old equipment needs to be replaced and new equipment needs to be purchased. Providers and their support personnel need to be well trained and paid. Facilities need to be maintained. And liability insurance needs to be purchased.

Many of these costs are not obvious in the day-to-day routine of medicine.

A patient visiting a doctor's office for a routine blood pressure check is unlikely to be aware of the x-ray machine in the back room, the chemistry laboratory down the hall, the room devoted to keeping medical records, or the personnel required to keep these functions operating.

There are nevertheless many costs that could be reduced particularly on bureaucratic side of healthcare. Government healthcare agencies are often overstocked with employees who engage in work of questionable value. Frequently, there are few incentives to get it right or to focus on the work one is supposed to do. Managers defend their positions in the status hierarchy, demand more employees, and shore up the defenses of their territories. Workers are often as concerned about their wages, the behavior of other employees, and the attitudes of management as they are about their jobs. Should a reader doubt these points, walk into any government healthcare facility and watch the way many individuals behave. Or telephone and try and obtain specific information. Should you call, one of four things will happen. First, you may spend half an hour pushing the buttons on your telephone. Next, after some button pushing, you may get to talk to a recorded voice that informs you that you are not calling during the correct business hours. Or again, after a period of button pushing, you may get to talk to someone who informs you that someone else needs to answer your question. This person promises to transfer your telephone call, which doesn't happen, and you start the process again. The final indignity is that the correct number, when identified, will be busy continually.

## LAWYERS AND MALPRACTICE

Any discussion about healthcare costs would be incomplete without considering malpractice. Malpractice suits against nearly every type of provider and institution involved in healthcare continue to proliferate, and they are a significant contributor to the rising cost of healthcare. In part, their high numbers are due to the unrealistic expectations of patients. Patients' desires need to be balanced against the fact that few patients are truly informed about the likely outcomes of medical care. In part, malpractice cases are due to low-quality healthcare, but in part they are an outgrowth of the predatory efforts of lawyers. Rather than participate in the improvement of healthcare, lawyers often actively impede improvement through the use of semantic manipulations and create doubt through innuendo.

Again, let us be clear on this point. In situations where providers or institutions have failed to meet reasonable medical standards or contractual responsibilities (e.g., HMOs and insurance companies), or where important medical information has been suppressed, as is apparently the case in the recent diet pill fiasco, legal action may be appropriate.[20,21] But this is a far cry from the world of frivolous law suits where, for example, 1 in 100,000 persons has a peculiar response to a drug or a dangerous surgery does not restore an individual to his or her predisease state.

## GOVERNMENT RESPONSES

Spurred by the public's complaints and findings from audits, the federal government has begun to act. As this chapter is being written, Congress is considering (a) mandating that managed care plans cover certain benefits such as emergency care and experimental treatments, (b) establishing procedures for independent appeals of decisions by managed care plans that deny benefits, and (c) requiring managed care plans to divulge information about their contracts with healthcare providers in their networks.[22] The president is advocating that persons 62 to 64 years of age be given the opportunity to pay for Medicare and is considering a "Patients' Rights" order. Congress is considering tough healthcare standards. States are also acting. California, for example, has devised a "Healthy Families" program to assure that children have access to healthcare—the catch is that the plan will cover only a percent of the children who need and do not have such care. The list of actual and proposed actions would take up at least another ten pages.

Often the federal and state rules that govern different facets of healthcare are in conflict. Often they are so complex that they are literally impossible to understand. Well-intentioned, proper and sensible behavior frequently turns out to be a violation of some law or guideline. In turn, time is wasted trying to address the complaints of regulators who live and die by the narrow interpretation of their rulebooks and have little sense of the context in which they are working. What are the upshots of these rules? They are these. There is often an inverse relationship between the intensity of regulation and the actual delivery of care. Laws, rules, and guidelines are an important cause for increased healthcare costs.

Still, one might reasonably ask, "If government rules and monitoring were eliminated, would not the quality of care decline?" In our current environment the answer is probably yes. There are other solutions to this problem, however, and these will be addressed later. Clearly, that government has a hand in healthcare is not necessarily bad. The issues are what type of influence it should have and how effectively it can use this influence. Medical licensing, establishing medical reeducation requirements, and setting and monitoring requirements for both the education and administration of highly technical procedures (e.g., PET) are activities where government participation would be useful. For these activities, standards that apply in Virginia and Montana can be expected to apply in Oregon and Louisiana. That is, it is possible to establish a uniform code or set of standards that have near universal applicability. On the other hand, when judg-

**Figure 4.2**
**Estimates in Dollars of Medicare and Medicaid Fraud Seizures between 1985 and 1997**

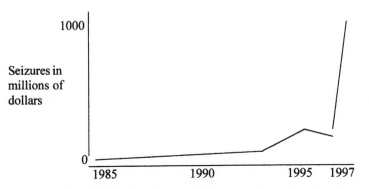

ment calls are involved—that is, when a physician is treating patients—it's best to leave government out of the picture.

## FRAUD

Fraud is almost always a factor when resources are involved. Healthcare, because it consumes so much of the US gross national product, turns out to be one of the prime arenas for fraudulent schemes. Figure 4.2 which shows estimates of the Medicare/Medicaid fraud seizures between 1985 and 1997, gives a hint of the prevalence of fraudulent medical billing, which some auditors believe is as high as 10%.[23]

Figure 4.2 illustrates an all-too-familiar picture. As the efforts of auditors have intensified, more and more questionable financial activities in healthcare have been found. But why? Like any other field, healthcare can be expected to have its percentage of persons who cheat. Yet this is only part of the problem. Payment systems (insurance, Medicare, Medicaid) that bring about longer working hours, an increasing percentage of time spent in unproductive work (paperwork and creating endless audit trails of one's activities), and declining benefits ratchet up the incentives for medical fraud.

Falsifying records about patient visits and treatment often occur at the level of the individual clinician. There is, however, another side to healthcare fraud that is conducted by organizations knowingly instituting fraudulent billing practices. One variation amounts to finding loopholes in existing rules or payments plans and exploiting them for profit in preference to providing care. Another is that hospitals create treatment annexes that are not subject to cost constraints or auditing that for most other healthcare services is a part of day-to-day life. Other groups have found that home healthcare is a lucrative way to avoid payment caps. Some organizations simply fail to exercise "due diligence" that bills are correct. Such practices are yet other entries on the list of perverse incentives.

It is hard to look at charts like Figure 4.2 and not be an advocate of strict healthcare monitoring (audits) and legal interventions. And once again for the record, we are advocates of the principle of monitoring. Yet an unfortunate fact of life is that the existing monitoring systems and the ongoing attempts to bring about legal remedies to healthcare are a part of the very system that needs to be corrected, not perpetuated. When law and regulation are impossible to understand, crime will flourish.

## HEALTHCARE—PATIENT CONTRIBUTIONS

Patients and patient interest groups are not innocent of contributing to the current state of healthcare. As we have pointed out several times, a percentage of patients have unrealistic expectations about what medicine can provide. When their expectations are not met, they become angry, often form advocacy groups, write their congressional representative, or hire lawyers. There is also the issue of rights. A large percentage of patients act on the assumption that both health and healthcare are rights. Disease-specific or other public interest groups spill into this category. Fueled by the belief that providers are inattentive to their concerns about a particular disease or disorder, they demand changes, hire influence peddlers, and initiate legislation. In turn, the healthcare picture becomes even more confused and resources that might be better spent elsewhere are often directed to meet their demands.

## CONCLUDING COMMENTS

We began this chapter with the question, "What is the state of the US healthcare system?" The quick answer is that it is a mess. That "mess" is an accurate term is suggested by President Clinton's proposal for a bill of rights for healthcare. His proposal is essentially a proclamation that patients should have certain protections, including equal treatment, regardless of their race or ethnicity, that patients can participate in treatment decisions, and that confidentiality of patient medical records is essential. Yet what does it mean when the president needs to propose a bill of rights for healthcare? In effect, the call for a bill of rights is a clear indication that our healthcare system is out of balance, there is little indication that it is improving, and that there are too many players in the healthcare arena.

There are other topics that we might have discussed in this chapter. The behavior of drug companies is an example. There are simply too many incidents like those recently reported for diet pill producers who did not pass on to the FDA early reports from Belgian doctors concerning the heart valve consequences of their drugs. There is the topic of our bodies being commercialized through the activities of HMOs, insurance companies, and the government. Then there is payment for psychotherapy. Many patients pay for their psychotherapy out of their own pockets because they fear what will happen if their HMOs or insurance companies have knowledge that they are seeking psychiatric care. There is also the topic of the increasing number of doctors attempting to work outside managed care.

Important as they are, these preceding topics pale in comparison to the basic underlying change during the last five decades of healthcare in the United States—somewhere between World War II and the present, when medicine moved from a service profession to an exploitive system.

## NOTES

1. Technology is frequently disparaged because of its putative cost enhancement. But there are many improvements we would not wish to do without. D. J. Weatherall reports in the *Times Literary Supplement*, 30 January 1988, for example, that clinical genetics holds remarkable promise for the future.

2. AIDS deaths have begun to decline in the United States, although not in Asia and Africa. In the *Wall Street Journal*, 28 February 1998, O. Suris discusses this development on the basis of a report from the Centers for Disease Control in Atlanta.

3. Conflict of interest among healthcare providers is a vexing problem. T. Burton, *Wall Street Journal*, 19 March 1998, discusses the confounding that develops when providers have a financial interest in the products they use.

4. I. Illich, *Medical Nemesis* (New York: Pantheon, 1976), p. 47.

5. See N. F. McKenzie (ed.), *Beyond Crisis* (New York: Meridian, 1994) as a source for many of the statistics developed here.

6. While it is always possible with figures of this type may be debatable because they depend upon judgment calls, it is generally recognized that there are too many unnecessary operations. See, for example, R. S. Mendelsohn, *Confessions of a Medical Heretic* (Chicago: Contemporary Books, 1979).

7. This is the predictable consequence of the currently operating incentives. See I. Fisher, *New York Times*, 11 January 1998, in which pending increases in HMO premiums are discussed.

8. Senior citizens represent an exception. M. Freudenheim, *New York Times*, 2 August 1997, reports that those over age 65 continue to join managed care plans at accelerated rates, largely because of expectations of lower costs and better benefits.

9. Stress on one part of the system is likely to strain another. G. Anders reports in the *Wall Street Journal*, 16 April 1998, that Medicare's austerity is easing an increasing number of the elderly into HMOs thought to be frugal.

10. Communication between physician and patient is important for many reasons, not the least of which is the avoidance of or timely treatment of adverse drug reactions. T. Monmaney reports in the *Los Angeles Times*, 15 April 1998, that between 76,000 and 137,000 people died in 1994 from this cause. More than 2 million had reactions requiring medical attention. Many of these reactions result from patients' attempts at self-medication.

11. Although the clinicians retain de jure authority, the de facto decisions are constrained by largely anonymous and unaccountable administrators. Liability has not made a similar transition. T. Bodenheimer, M D, and K. Sullivan, J D, *New England Journal of Medicine*, 9 April 1998, discuss how large employers are shaping the healthcare marketplace through their close attention to expenses.

12. Disconnection between responsibility and decision making encourages disjunction between promised care and its actual delivery. See A. J. Rubin, *Los Angeles Times*, 19 November 1997, for a discussion of the so-called "Healthcare Bill of Rights" recommended by a presidential commission as a remedy for this power imbalance. We reserve the right to retain skepticism that more laws and regulations will have a salubrious effect.

13. But this is by no means the only problem. See G. Anders and E. Rodriguez, "Never Mind the Fraud: What Ails Medicare Is Often Perfectly Legal," *Wall Street Journal*, 9 October 1997, in which they discuss some of the ways hospitals develop annexes and push home healthcare to avoid payment caps.

14. If we wish to get a good look at the future, one of the most useful tools is to examine the structure of incentives. See, for example, S. Simon, in *Los Angeles Times*, 8 December 1998. The author discusses California's proposed "Health Families" legislation, which would provide health insurance to low-income families. This legislation seems to hold mixed promise. The article illustrates how the best of intentions can get lost when politics enters the picture.

15. So it would seem that a fine line must be drawn for organizational survival—be competitive, even ruthless, but avoid being greedy. See A. Rubin, *Los Angeles Times* 14 January 1998, for coverage of Congressional efforts to pass legislation to ensure protection for consumers when they deal with managed care companies.

16. A. Rubin outlines the many proposed "cures" for managed care problems being considered by Congress in the *Los Angeles Times*, 22 October 1997.

17. R. Rosenblatt reports in the *Los Angeles Times*, 4 December 1997, of a survey which revealed that 42% of patients with health insurance in 1996 had problems with their coverage; 13% of California patients enrolled in Medicare HMOs quit their plans each year. Interestingly, the author sees 13% as a low dropout rate and believes that the figure represents a significant level of satisfaction in the elderly.

18. The HMOs are nevertheless usually able to raise their fees. Consider a report by D. Olmos in the *Los Angeles Times*, 1 April 1998, which describes a planned 11% increase in rates for Kaiser Permanente, the nation's largest healthcare provider.

19. See *USA Today*, 6 August 1997.

20. For example, consider an article by L. Johannes and S. Stecklow in the *Wall Street Journal*, 11 December 1997. They document how American sellers of diet pills heard reports from Belgium about potential heart valve problems but passed on only some of this information to the Food and Drug Administration.

21. See R. Schmitt, *Wall Street Journal*, 8 January 1998. Judges are beginning to worry that class-action lawsuits can inflate legal costs at the expense of payment to persons suffering damage. The concerns address the 6 million people who may be worried about heart valve and lung disease associated with diet pills.

22. See M. Moss and C. Adams, *Wall Street Journal*, 7 April 1998. The authors point out how Medicaid patients are being abandoned by big HMO firms in some states after having extracted as much money as possible.

23. See *USA Today*, 6 August 1997.

*Part II*

# What Key Healthcare Players Want

*Chapter 5*

# What Patients Want

---

> You would think that they could organize this place to take account of patients. . . . I've been here three hours, waiting for a routine blood pressure check. . . . The appointment was at 10 A.M. . . . It didn't stop the docs from having lunch or glancing at the sports page. . . . I could excuse it if it didn't happen regularly. . . . I'm searching for somewhere else to get my care.
>
> Conversation with an insured patient
> in the waiting room of a large HMO

## INTRODUCTION

What patients want medically depends on their condition at the time they are asked. When patients are healthy, they want convenience, comfort, and reassurance with negligible out-of-pocket expenses. The situation changes when they are seriously ill or injured. At such times they want prompt attention, restoration of health, and, if possible, comfort. They hope for wise and confident caregivers, insisting that no effort be spared and no possibility overlooked in the quest for their return to health. They have no patience with the idea that persons other than their caretakers might decide how much care they need or what kind of care they receive. Out-of-pocket costs are of less concern—people are usually willing to bear great expense to restore their own health or that of their loved ones.

Most of the care that is delivered goes to the sick. Yet, currently, a large percentage of the decisions about healthcare delivery is made by healthy people, many of whom have difficulty imagining that their perspectives might change if they became ill. Thus, it is not entirely surprising that there are major areas of disagreement about our current healthcare delivery system as well as future systems on the drawing board. For example, healthcare delivery experts and economists often note that an unusually large percentage of healthcare expenses are incurred during the last year of life. One wonders why such statements are made. Is it because healthcare costs would decline if we shortened the final year of our lives? Probably not. Or is it because such statements are made by healthcare planners who are healthy and who are analyzing the cost figures without consideration of their implications. Probably. What seems to escape the notice of these planners is that healthcare during the last year of life is expensive because it is then that most people are seriously ill. More important, for most persons, there is no way of knowing beforehand whether one has entered that last expensive year.

Who are the patients? We are *all* patients! Alas, this obvious fact it is not always clear. Nurses and physicians, lawyers and clients, elected officials, career civil servants, insurance company executives and their staffs, professors and students, liberals and conservatives—all are patients whether they recognize it nor not. Viewed this way, all of us have an equal interest in having a system of healthcare delivery that is rational and humane from the perspective of the recipient of care. Rational and humane delivery is not necessarily what occurs, however. Our capacity to deny illness is well studied, if not always fully understood. Less well examined is our power to deny that we will ever get sick. Nevertheless, decisions by the major healthcare payers and planners are often made without having incorporated this insight into their thinking.[1]

Left to themselves, a sizable percentage of healthcare planners (e.g., planners working for HMOs, insurance companies, the government, charitable institutions) have been unable to imagine better alternative healthcare solutions than the ones currently in place. This is not surprising. Planners are usually immersed in efforts to solve cost-delivery equations, or they are tinkering with minor cost-benefit glitches in the current system. In fairness to these planners, the cost of healthcare is an important consideration. Yet it is, finally, ancillary to the main point of care: cure, if possible, and at very least, improvement of a medical condition. Patients who come from different social, cultural, and economic backgrounds may disagree about the amenities of healthcare, but all agree that the beginning of wisdom in healthcare is that improvement in the patient's condition is the whole point of the exercise. The amenities mean nothing unless this prime directive is kept firmly in mind.

The purpose of healthcare is not to elect politicians, not to provide employment for accountants, not to enlarge or enrich insurance companies, not to increase the influence of government, not to provide dividends for the stockholders, not to sell pharmaceuticals, not to build hospitals and clinics, and not to overly enhance the incomes of providers. Still, as health-care decision making has progressively passed out of the purview of the patient, it has fallen like a ripe plum into the agendas of impersonal planners and institutions. Examine the financial pages of national newspapers if you doubt this point. When insurance companies are evaluated for their financial health and suitability for investment, the major thrust of the article addresses the potential for profit. Up to a point, this is fine. What is not fine is that such articles seldom address the human costs that accompany the desire for profit. An insurance company is considered a good investment to the extent that it is able to minimize its "medical losses"—medical loss is the industry's technical term for care actually delivered. In effect, the agenda is to increase cash flow by charging as much as possible and delivering as little as possible. Insurance companies are able to get away with such strategies, in large part, because their clients are unaware of the details of medicine and alternative options for delivery. Yet, clearly, such strategies are not stable in the long run. And because they are not, our healthcare system is continually in a state of turmoil.

That financial institutions have profit as their main concern is neither surprising nor inappropriate. Successful institutions are what we hope to have. Nor are we advocating that insurance companies, HMOs, and the like pour all their assets into our idea of quality healthcare and then enter bank-ruptcy. The point is otherwise. What must be kept firmly in mind is that we as patients cannot abdicate healthcare policy decisions to for-profit institu-tions. Why? Because their inherent nature compels them to have priorities that are not central to what should be healthcare's main mission—to cure or, at least, to improve. Nor should we single out financial institutions as villains. Professional associations, building contractors, pharmaceutical com-panies, etc., have vested interests and priorities that are natural, understand-able, and legal. But we need to recognize that their institutional incentives are not necessarily the same as those of patients. In short, if patients do not regain the operational control of the healthcare rule-making and resource-allocating process, no other group is likely to do it right.

As the for-profit side of healthcare has assumed a larger portion of the healthcare dollar, government has found itself increasingly drawn into the service delivery arena in order to limit perceived abuses, to audit, and to require that certain standards are met. It is hard to question the intentions of such actions—many are necessary; however, it is less hard to question the consequences. New laws, new rules, and more healthcare audits by FBI agents do not necessarily equate with improved healthcare. For example, there is little indication that medical fraud is declining despite the rising number of convictions for bilking insurance companies, Medicare, and Med-icaid. Some insurance company profits are increasing and some are in de-cline, some HMOs are getting bigger and some are going out of business and, most importantly, neither the availability of care nor the quality of care is improving. Unfortunately, government's participation adds to the confusion and delays any resolution of the problems in our healthcare system.

To rephrase some of the key points above, when we are sick, we are not "clients." Nor do we wish to consider ourselves as consumers or members of a healthcare organization. We want quality care in a timely fashion and at reasonable cost. It follows that the design of our healthcare system should reflect what we want when we are sick. It is serious illness that sharpens our discernment of quality. This brings us to specific healthcare delivery modes as they are viewed from the perspective of the sick individual.

## THE FEE-FOR-SERVICE DELIVERY MODE

The fee-for-service mode will be considered first. In this variation of healthcare delivery, patients enjoy supreme autonomy. They pay for the advice of their providers, and the advice patients receive is usually directed towards their expressed requests. There is always the possibility that providers will misdiagnose an illness, or that they will act in self-interested ways by recommending more extensive or expensive treatment than might be necessary. Yet the patient is free to inquire in detail whether this might be so and take such action as seems to be indicated, such as to obtain a second opinion. In effect, providers in this mode may not be perfectly disinterested agents, but they are without a doubt the agents of the patient. Allowing that diagnoses are likely to be correct, the major disadvantages of this mode have to do with cost. The patient may pay for unnecessary evaluation and treatment, or she or he may forgo necessary care in order to avoid incurring expenses that seem to be overpriced.

Other criticisms of the fee-for-service mode tend to question the efficiency of privately contracted care. Patients may ask for treatment that they do not need, and physicians might agree to provide it. All people, even when they become patients, place different value on certain intangibles such as degree of pain, the importance of timely treatment, and the courtesy with which the care is delivered. Fee-for-service providers generally respond to these values. Of course, planners are always eager to make such allocation decisions because in their view they know what is best for patients. Their decisions often miss the mark, however, because they overlook the fact that there are many possible ways to measure quality of care and patient satisfaction. For example, both quality of care and patient satisfaction can improve when patients exercise informed choices. Although such choices may be biased, these biases can average out if a wary patient consults more than one provider.

## INDEMNITY INSURANCE

As noted, comprehensive insurance to defray the cost of medical care became an important economic fact during World War II, a period in which people were not accustomed to having routine medical care as a standard feature of their lives. As the decades passed, more medical procedures became available. In turn, expectations of regular medical visits increased. As they did, the rationale for funding through an indemnity insurance mechanism became less tenable. Indemnity insurance only makes sense when the events for which it is designed are unusual, and when actuarial calculations and estimates of risk can be applied. Insurance to pay the costs for events that are certain to occur is inefficient and ultimately unstable. Despite the fine print of insurance policies, patients expect the coverage they believe they deserve because they have paid an insurance premium. In fiscal self-defense, insurance companies have found it necessary to assert the right to disapprove certain expenses as unnecessary. As they have done this, a spiral of perverse incentives ensues, causing a tangle of misunderstanding among patients, providers, and insurers.

## MEDICARE AND MEDICAID

Although these government-supported plans were designed to provide care for the elderly, disabled, and indigent, they suffer from many of the same perverse incentives that plague indemnity insurance plans. There is the added difficulty that the costs and benefits of these plans are subject to the political process, which allows for still greater excursions of cost and provision of care. The federal and state governments, having both the ability to tax and to generate greater cash reserves than the healthiest of insurance companies, can subsidize vastly greater inefficiencies than any insurance company can tolerate and still remain fiscally solvent. Yet even the government has its fiscal limits. As healthcare expenditures have become unsustainable, there have been efforts to try to control costs by hidden or explicit price controls, or by the passage of laws that define the level of medical care each citizen may have.

When it comes to laws defining level of care, stop a moment and ask the following question: "What kinds of assumptions guide such decisions?" The answer is not hard to come by: not only does the government assume that it knows how much care individuals need, but also what type of care should be provided. In effect, it assumes that it owns your body.[2] There is political pressure to make these decisions fair—that is, no one should have greater access to healthcare on the basis of financial circumstances, sex, age, or ethnicity. Again, all well and good. Still, when government enters the healthcare arena, the outcome is as often increased confusion, poor resolution, and little progress. Power tends to create the illusion of knowledge.[3]

## THE MANAGED CARE ENVIRONMENT

The basic underlying assumption of managed care programs is that there can be a single standard of medical care which can be understood and implemented, with negligible modification for individual differences. With profit the most important priority of corporate policy, there is an unavoidable tendency to draw up protocols that direct care with increasing stringency. This point applies equally to so-called "nonprofit" institutions. Such protocols, or "care maps," purport to represent state-of-the-art care for each diagnosis. Unfortunately, when final authority for such maps is invested in a corporate manager, the details of care must finally be compatible with the expected earnings. Physicians may indeed design these treatment strategies initially, but corporate policy has the power to alter them as fiscal constraints may require. Thus, there is an incentive to ratchet down the actual care delivered. Because the recipients of the managed care services—patients— would prefer to think that their care has some relation to their individual needs, progressively greater efforts at obfuscation and deception are employed. In this scenario, the managed care company does not own your body, but perhaps it rents it. And it reserves the right to decide the definition of your care.[4]

## VETERINARY MEDICINE

Another style of care that has received very little attention or debate in the quest for healthcare clarity is veterinary medicine. Examination of this style of delivery is illuminating. The veterinary mode of care enjoyed by our pets and domestic animals generally is of very high quality. It usually employs the most advanced technology. The major difference is that animals have no decision autonomy and they must accept whatever procedures their owners desire. As these decisions are mostly benevolent, this system works well. There is another important feature of this style of care that deserves attention, namely that care is widely available at a small fraction of the costs incurred in human healthcare. This phenomenon of lower cost is well worth studying because in the United States the fee-for-service system is used for veterinary medicine, and regulatory burden is smaller.

Attempts at achieving high-quality care for humans while using the assumptions of veterinary medicine have been tried in certain venues. All that is necessary is to make explicit is that the patient has no decision autonomy; another authority will assume the position of healthcare guardian. In the United States, this style has been used in the military service, generally during wartime. In noncritical times, the military member may elect privately contracted care, while being responsible for some or all of the costs. Thus, such care is not totally binding. Where it is, other issues arise. For example, Cuba has been the most energetic exemplar of the veterinary care model in recent years. Healthcare is universal, and without direct cost to all Cubans. However, decisions remain the exclusive prerogative of the government, and quality is constrained by the exigencies of current economic development.

Decision autonomy at the level of the patient is expensive. Americans need to come to an agreement about how much autonomy we want to buy. We also need to settle whether our decision will be collective and binding on all of us, or whether each citizen might select a style of healthcare delivery that is congruent with the value each places on this autonomy.

## WE WANT QUALITY OF CARE

Quality of care has several dimensions, and each is measured in units that are not commensurate. As noted, how we define quality changes with the circumstances of our health—the unavoidable truth is that quality has a different meaning to us when we are healthy than when we are sick. Until the problems inherent in the measurement of quality are widely recognized, there will be endless non-productive debate on the issue.

To review, when we are healthy, our views of quality have a lot to do with comfort, convenience, and accessibility. Considerations include access to a provider by means of an early appointment or even a walk-in service as long as the wait is short. We are not particularly concerned about the physician's skill if all we need is a form to be filled out or an influenza shot. At such moments we do not want quibbling, complications, or bad news. Rather, we tend to judge quality by the ambiance of the office, the courtesy with which we are received, the compliance with which our requests are viewed, and the charging of a small fee. In effect, we want to be treated as if we are the only patient to be seen that day. A system that would provide this kind of quality is of course possible, although not necessarily cheap. The problem is that treatment as if we are the only patient would be incompatible with other ideas of quality. Compromise is essential for a viable healthcare system. Yet compromise is not what we're thinking about when we're healthy, and it is when we are healthy that the majority of our healthcare selection decisions are made.

Next comes the question of quality under circumstances of routine care for mild or self-limiting illness. Here, we are concerned with the skill of our professionals, but we also want the intangibles, many of which filter up from childhood memories. We want providers with courage, compassion, and good humor to help us face discomfort and inconvenience. We also want the capacity for thoughtful diagnosis, judicious treatment, and a favorable prognosis. We expect accessibility for periodic reassurance. For mild or self-limiting illness, the physician should be equally skillful with children and adults, men and women, the young and the elderly. It should be possible to handle the great majority of healthcare problems in this way and without excessive cost. In the rare event that we have some condition of a serious or dangerous nature, we expect our providers to know when to refer us and to facilitate the transfer with a minimum of logistic difficulty or inconvenience.

Emergency care comes next. Quality in this venue has one salient dimension—speed. Not everything we imagine to be an emergency is necessarily life-threatening or otherwise in need of immediate intervention. The objective reality is not what counts, however. If we think a problem is an emergency, then we are likely to define quality in terms of the system's capacity to deal with it in a rapid and definitive manner. We are of course happy to hear that the chest pain we had was not a heart attack, but we still want the information delivered in an expeditious manner. Even good news delivered without proper appreciation for our concern does not indicate quality. Again, we want the costs not to be burdensome. We recognize that emergency care is likely to be expensive. When the emergency is our fault, we are more willing to tolerate a high bill than when it we are innocent. When it is due to the behavior of someone else, a high bill becomes more troublesome.

More serious is the problem of defining quality when we are very sick. Any rational calculus would suggest that this is the time when decisions about quality are most important, but because of the relative infrequency of major illnesses, we tend to avoid decisions concerning quality at that time. In this circumstance we want the most knowledgeable providers and the highest state-of-the-art in technology for the best diagnosis and treatment. And we want these services delivered with all due speed. Moreover, within limits, cost be damned, although it would be best if it were covered by some means other than out-of-pocket.

Where does this discussion of quality lead? In our view, it leads only one place: above all, and regardless of circumstances, we want to avoid "healthcare rationing." We must recognize that healthcare rationing is a term that means not only artificial control of supply and demand; it also can mean unacceptable constraints on efforts to find the best compromise of the three key variables of healthcare delivery: quality, accessibility, and cost. If these three variables are to be optimized, compromise we must. The important question is not whether to compromise, but how to design a system that places the priorities where they belong—saving lives comes first, routine care comes second, and lastly come ambiance and convenience. Said another way, we have to get used to the idea that quality measures might best be designed from the perspective of serious illness.

## WE WANT TRUSTWORTHY CAREGIVERS

Trust is a rare quality even in the best of times. Over the past few centuries professions have developed with the goal of delivering service in an ethical manner. To assure ethical standards, attorneys, physicians, engineers, educators and others who offer service to the public have banded together in professional associations and developed standards of probity and honor. Professions have come to be defined by three criteria: sapiential authority, fiduciary responsibility, and self-governance.

Sapiential authority refers to the capacity to give authoritative advice on the basis of detailed and comprehensive mastery of a segment of practical knowledge. It implies that a professional knows the limits of his or her skills and will refrain from attempts at practice outside these boundaries. The authority is based on factual knowledge and on observation and logic. It has been methodically developed as a consensus within the profession. It does not depend on faith-based presumptions, myths, or hopes. Statements are true to the extent that they correspond to empirically based and accumulated knowledge. Sapiential authority grows out of the Enlightenment insight that facts derive from evidence and not from the ascribed status of the speaker. This is, of course, an ideal that no profession has fully achieved. Professionals are humans first, with the usual self-interested motives and faults. Yet the concept remains, and the goal is ever pursued: find out the truth, and use it to the benefit of the client.

Fiduciary responsibility refers to the requirement that professionals stand in a special relationship of trust to the client. Professionals are expected to place the well-being of the client before their own financial interest for the duration of their contractual agreement. This means that the attorney must not generate unnecessary litigation, and the physician must not identify spurious illness for the purpose of inflating fees. Again, this ideal is not always fully adhered to, but it remains the goal and standard by which practitioners can be measured.

The third support on which professionalism stands is that of self-governance. While no profession or other association may justly operate beyond the limits of the civil law, there is nevertheless a responsibility to define the standards of expected conduct and knowledge within their profession and to determine which applicants meet these requirements. The profession, in collective assembly, may thus admit or expel members subject to the requirements for due process and fairness that the law requires.

The three traditional pillars of professionalism represent a set of ideals to which all members properly aspire and to which all clients have a right to expect. Yet, as we have and will argue, each has been eroded in recent years by a combination of governmental action and corporate profit-seeking. For example, with considerable success, HMOs have increasingly sought to assert sovereignty over the interpretation of medical knowledge. As a matter of policy, HMOs decide when certain tests are indicated, as well as the criteria for diagnoses. Some treatments receive the imprimatur as an appropriate use of corporate resources, while others are effectively forbidden.

Fiduciary responsibility has experienced similar atrophy. From the time of the invention of money until the present day, it has been clear that the one who controls financial resources is the one who controls the destiny of others. When patients are beguiled into thinking that the government or the corporation is paying for their care, they abandon any expectation that the physician is working for them. When patients realize that their own resources that are being used, they become more vigilant and insist that they be used wisely and in concert with their wishes. Still, fiduciary responsibility is a quality of character that may adhere only to individual professionals—when government or corporate institutions make a pretense to embrace it, their efforts are easily seen to be wanting.

Self-governance has also undergone metamorphosis. Peer review has never been fully effective in the achievement of complete honesty among physicians (and "alternative" means of medical care have been wholly outside any sanction peer review may have). Unfortunately, the action of government has effectively preempted the self-correcting professional impulse. Medical schools now shape their student bodies and their curricula in ways that meet with federal approval—it is hard to envision another outcome once one accepts the king's shilling. Managed care companies have begun to assert that their corporate principles should be at the core of the teaching process. Should these principles conflict with current scientific understanding, then science must understand and give way. In addition, healthcare corporations are increasingly asserting their power to decide who will work as a physician. The primary means they employ is their power to judge the credentials of caregivers periodically which, simply translated, means that HMOs can deny credentials to those who fail to meet the goals of corporate economic policy.[5]

## WE WANT AUTONOMY

Humans are by nature gregarious. We are immersed in social systems which have been, since the beginning of our species, essential to our individual survival. In today's world, a human being without the support and fellowship of kin and friends is hardly likely to be successful. (Isolated people in Paleolithic times were sentenced to certain death from predators, the elements, or enemies.) Nevertheless, self-autonomy remains not only a biological fact, but also one of the core values of free people. Each individual has a sovereignty over his body, while retaining a wish and an obligation for social connection.

Access to information about the nature of our bodies, and the means by which treatment may be accomplished, is at the core of a successful system of healthcare. Patients need to know about some of the details of patho-physiology, the reputations of those responsible for their care, the means by which the quality of their treatment may be assessed, and the integrity of the institutions employed for their care. One of the traditional roles of the provider is to instruct the patient in health and disease. In the modern world, however, it is necessary to augment this duty with an explanation of the rules and incentives that pervade the systems of delivery currently in fashion. Although such explanations are in the patient's best interest, the free flow of information is often derided by the modern healthcare executive. Following the model that truth is whatever best suits the strongest, some corporate authorities have invented the "gag rule," by which physicians are sanctioned if they provide patients with frank assessments of their healthcare plan or if they inform the patient of therapeutic options that might reduce profit maximization. Fortunately, courts have begun to void such restrictions, but the process will be long, the battle intense, and the corrective means inefficient.[6]

Autonomy requires making a choice of healthcare providers. To be meaningful, this choice must be among providers with more than one point of view. It is a not a real choice when a patient is given a long list of names of physicians, all required to conform to corporate policy decisions. The critical element is that the physician or other provider be allowed to act as the agent of the patient. Most HMOs advertise that choice of physicians is preserved within their plan, but virtually without exception, this choice is constrained in ways that serve corporate policy. This represents another example of the illusion that professionals may be considered as interchangeable parts. The situation is similar to a supermarket advertising a choice of soups, and yet the shelves are stocked with choices all made by the same company differing only in their labels.

When a patient protests that the idea of choice is spurious, the HMO manager or the insurance company representative usually points out that the patient does have a choice of a long list of providers which she or he may consult. Such discussions leave out one key point: the choice of providers, in order to be meaningful, implies the patient's power to refuse care from anyone who fails to earn and keep his or her trust. This in turn requires that physicians retain considerable decision autonomy. Failing that, in an HMO environment, there must be a robust choice of companies, which is only the case if one is healthy at the time. Autonomy implies the patient's right to control the therapeutic process throughout the course of the illness. Physicians can advise, and companies can confirm or deny payment, but autonomy is not meaningful if, for personal reasons, the patient wishes to have treatment proceed along a course different from that recommended. Should the course not be congruent with good practice, the physician must be free to withdraw as well.

As in every other aspect of our healthcare desires, autonomy is an ideal that must be considered within a broad matrix of compromise. Perfect autonomy implies a perfectly free market and advanced knowledge of the product one is purchasing—conditions that hardly exist anywhere, even for the simplest of products. Autonomy thus must be placed in the context of other competing values. We will never have a system, nor should we, wherein there is no government regulation, no payment through third parties, and no economic constraints. Still, autonomy is a critical consideration. Unless this ideal is kept at the forefront of our minds, there will never be a system that is congruent with historical American assumptions and values.[7]

Time and again we have asked, "Who owns our bodies?" Time and again we have answered, "We do—each of us individually." Not the government, not "humanity," not the insurance company, and certainly not healthcare providers. If individual rights and civil liberties mean anything, then it should be clear that we can all agree on this basic starting point. This means having the right to make contracts freely with providers for services. It means having fair review in the courts for the government's administrative actions that impact on our families. It means controls or limits on the extent to which outside parties may intrude on our privacy. It means strong protection for confidentiality. It means curbs on information flow concerning testing for genetic diseases. It means that diagnosis and treatment must be individualized—the clinical arts do not flourish in a "cookie cutter" or a "paint-by-numbers" environment. Finally, it means that there are substantial reasons to cooperate as good citizens for the establishment of proper public health measures. Autonomy and connection are with us to stay.

## WE WANT EASY ACCESS TO CARE

In recent years a variety of encumbrances have intruded into the delivery of healthcare. Control and limitation of payments by insurance companies and government have induced apparent shortages of providers. Complex regulation of the referral process, frequent and unannounced changes in rules and procedures, and retroactive unilateral denial of payments without effective appeal have all contributed to patients' frustration and anger. For routine healthcare, we want the convenience of a location near our homes. We presume, usually correctly, that most of the usually medical problems can be managed well by most physicians, and so a search for one who is supremely qualified is unnecessary. We expect convenient hours, appointments without too much delay, and short waiting times. Courtesy of the supporting staff is an important consideration. Access to parking or public transportation is expected as well.

On the other hand, there are times when only the best will do. As we have noted, for serious illnesses, we expect efficient referral to tertiary centers (generally, large hospitals with many providers) where every advancement in technology is available and professionals have the most up-to-date training. Usually such centers are located in large urban centers and affiliated with medical schools. These are usually centers of ongoing research, and as such we seldom mind being "guinea pigs" as long as this insures the most modern and "cutting edge" treatment. We will tolerate a bit of brusqueness and inconvenience, but we expect that our providers will be at the top of the ladder of professional competence.

Similar principles apply to emergency care. In emergencies, we want it all, including short travel distance, no waiting, instant and accurate diagnostic assessment, and rapid, effective, curative treatment. In these circumstances we expect that our health plan will be flexible enough to allow for distinctions among routine, tertiary, and emergency care. We expect that a well-functioning web of services will match our needs and do so with a minimum of bureaucratic impediments.

## WE WANT CONFIDENTIALITY

As the science and technology of medicine has advanced relentlessly, more and more aspects of our lives have become entangled with it. At one time, confidentiality was not too difficult to achieve because medical capability was limited; therefore, the number of private and potentially embarrassing pieces of information was small. In the modern era, however, greater capacity for information storage and retrieval, enhanced preventive capability, a greater spectrum of therapeutic choices, and widely based diagnostic screening have all caused a movement toward vastly greater amounts of personal data to be safeguarded.

As the technology of therapeutics has advanced, so has the technology of intrusiveness. Employers who pay for care as a fringe benefit have an interest in knowing those medical conditions that might plausibly impinge on job performance. When employers pay, there is a natural tendency to assume that they should have access to relevant data. Earlier we noted that many persons receiving psychotherapy pay out-of-pocket for fear of the consequences should the fact of their treatment become known at corporate levels. To be sure, the pretense of voluntary consent is preserved. No one has the right to see your medical record without your consent. Nevertheless, this consent is usually easily obtained by the implicit or explicit threat to terminate employment.

Similarly, insurance companies routinely assert their right to know everything about you that is contained in medical records—and these days, records can contain quite a lot indeed. Included may be evidence of psychiatric illness or consultation, alcohol or drug abuse, marital disharmony, genetic vulnerability to disease, chronic illness that might shorten life, medications taken and their expected side effects and, of course, the whole spectrum of venereal disease. In short, there is a potential for exposure of a huge array of embarrassments which can cause idiosyncratic management decisions.

Consent for release of medical information is routinely asked for and received by employers and insurance companies. This consent usually contains the provision that the information and the consent may be passed along to others with a "need to know," which may be very broadly construed. Thus, by signing a permission for access to our records we are, in fact, granting what amounts to a license to explore our most intimate concerns by a vast army of functionaries, not all of whom will be scrupulous. As information processing capacities for easy access and transfer continue to be enhanced, hopes for any meaningful privacy further decay.

What is to be done? There is but one way to guarantee a reasonable level of confidentiality. Recognizing that no way is perfect, the best we can do is to limit access to the information to those who have a fiduciary obligation to us—that is, the professionals who take personal responsibility for our care. Only they can be held accountable for any malfeasance associated with improper disclosure.

Yet how can we deny access to those who have the capacity to coerce us? Again, there is but one way. If confidentially is really important to us, then we must be the ones who pay the professionals. At one stroke, this removes any claim of a "need to know" by any fiscal intermediaries. True, the world is full of busybodies who would know our medical histories in order to take better care of us, but without a monetary excuse, these can be controlled without too much difficulty.

## WE WANT COHERENCE IN FAMILY CARE

As the complexity of medical care has increased there has been a tendency to divide delivery along the lines of age and sex. This makes some sense from the point of view of the medical specialist who prefers to concentrate on a limited set of pathologic conditions. Nevertheless, it can cause considerable logistic difficulty for a multigenerational family. There are neonatologists, pediatricians—adolescent physicians, general internists, gynecologists, and geriatricians—and that is just the beginning. A wide variety of specialists cut across these lines, and most families encounter a number of them. Dentists and dermatologists, allergists and ophthalmologists, psychiatrists and orthopedists, all make up the great orchestra in the symphony of medical care for the average modern family.

That so much specialization exists is in part a testament to the complexity and depth of knowledge and skill that we expect; as a rule, we tolerate confusion, however irritating it may be. Another modern factor adds further distress—payment methods are often different for each of the groups and specialties. Medicare covers those over age 65 whether they want it or not. For many conditions, many HMOs consider certain specialties as elective. Some insurance plans cover certain conditions and exclude others, depending on age or tenure. Some routine procedures and preexisting conditions are not covered. Some procedures considered experimental are not covered even though they may represent state-of-the-art care. Furthermore, any and all of these rules and guidelines may be changed—frequently, unilaterally, and without notice—by a third-party payer. Such a chaotic system invites passivity in patients and providers alike. When a family must confront an incoherent system of healthcare that provides different benefits and rules through different third-party payers to each member, multigenerational care is thwarted. A cacophony of demands and requirements from governments and corporations thus fails to nurture family harmony and cohesiveness. A more satisfactory system would allow for all members of the family to be treated with substantial equity.

## WE WANT REASONABLE COSTS

This topic is about "affordability," yet to use that term is to distort the issue. The first thing that must be recognized is that *we* are the actual payers in whatever system we may devise. Politicians, insurance companies, and providers may occasionally attempt to divert our attention from this obvious fact. Yet we will make no progress in our healthcare systems until we accept the fact that, whatever values and resources are directed to healthcare, the costs come from our pockets. The question is whether it is better to pay the costs directly by savings or indirectly through the intermediation of government or insurance.

Reasonable people may differ on the best way to solve this dilemma. Ideally, we might have a system so flexible that either option might be available for our choice. Each has advantages and disadvantages. Thus, we must examine this decision with respect to the capacity of each method to provide a stable system that will satisfy as many of the other desirable healthcare criteria as possible.

Indirect payments (e.g., insurance company, HMO) provide some comfort in that the payments we make are generally automatic. We do not have to take responsibility for making decisions to allocate resources or make budgets. With indirect payments, we can expect somewhat more uniformity in the style of care. There will be a more complex regulatory environment that will tend to produce more stable and predictable results. We never see the money used, so we do not learn to miss it, and we do not have to make difficult decisions about whether to use the money in other ways. Although we lose direct control of our care because we lack economic leverage, we can still influence the process by political activity, or by resort to litigation.

On the other side of the coin, indirect payments cause us to trade autonomy and control for security and uniformity. Administrative costs, whether incurred by government or the private sector, can amount to a substantial fraction of the total expenditure. Confidentiality becomes much more problematic with indirect payment. Incentives are skewed to limit easy access to preferred providers.

At last, the question is reduced to that most ancient of political dilemmas: "Which is more important, freedom or equality?" We are firmly aware that this question is not likely to be finally settled here. We prefer freedom, yet we recognize that all may not concur. To those who do not concur, we need to demonstrate that the choice of the freedom of direct payment is consistent with a stable, high-quality, self-correcting system that has tolerable costs for the average family. Because not all will agree that direct payment is desirable (even if it is possible), we need to be sufficiently flexible to allow for the choice of indirect payment as well for those who wish it, or those whose income makes direct payment infeasible.

But how would direct payment be accomplished? Could we afford it? Would we freedom-lovers be sufficiently responsible to be sure our care ·would be adequately planned and funded in advance? Would we take appropriate preventive measures? Would public health initiatives be compromised? Would there be adequate safeguards to avoid unscrupulous use of ineffective treatment?

In the abstract, we can afford direct payment. Indeed, we are affording it. True, transfer payments and cross-subsidization mean that some of us pay more than others, but in the aggregate the costs of direct payment will be lower than indirect payment, because administrative costs will be lower and market discipline will be more effective. We live in the real world, however, not in the abstract. How could it work?

First, we will need to limit "out-of-pocket" costs. But whence comes money if not from pockets? The answer is that it comes from two sources: medical savings accounts and insurance as reimbursement for unexpected or catastrophic illness.

Medical savings accounts are already being tried in a small pilot program. They are like an Individual Retirement Account into which we place the money we would otherwise pay as insurance premiums. These funds would be tax-deductible, and mandatory if the program were elected. They would be invested such that the benefits of compound interest could be brought into play. The money could be used only for medical costs. In the usual case, most of the costs of care occur at advanced age, when the account would be most robust.

Still, there are times when the young get very sick, and the elderly may likewise suffer an illness which exhausts the capacity of the account. For this contingency, a "catastrophic" insurance policy is appropriate. It would be cheap compared to currently available indemnity or managed care plans which attempt to cover all types of care delivery. And it would reimburse the patient for costs he or she has already found to be worthy of incurring. In turn, market discipline would be retained.

Best of all, a combination of medical savings accounts and catastrophic insurance would get the insurance companies out of the unenviable position of pretending to be direct providers of medical care, a task for which they have no expertise. Insurance would return to its original and proper function, that of sharing financial risk in case of unusual misfortune. At best, they could offer a flexible series of combined plans, each crafted for age and special circumstances.

## WE WANT A CHOICE OF PROVIDERS AND PAYMENT METHODS

Any system that attempts to solve all problems will in the end be seen to satisfy no one. Living in a society of increasing diversity of opinion, we expect increasing freedom of individual choice. That the United States, alone among industrialized countries, has thus far avoided a single standard and single payer for healthcare is strongly suggestive evidence that uniformity is not among the most salient of our values.

Recognizing that there is an unavoidable conflict between the values of autonomy and equality, we can hope for a system that is characterized by flexibility and compromise. The free market can leave some people behind, while a uniform system of government care brings equality at too high a price to suit most Americans. Having insurance companies deliver healthcare brings about the disadvantages of both. We can now search for a way to bring substantial equality together with substantial freedom of choice.

## NOTES

1. The argument is sometimes made that patient dissatisfaction can be alleviated by having a choice of providers. But G. Annas of Boston University, writing in the *New England Journal of Medicine*, 17 July 1997, has pointed out that this does not guarantee that rights will be preserved or that quality will improve. Choice among insurance plans that share essential basic assumptions may be no choice at all.

2. Consider, for example, the policy of the Health Care Finance Administration, well described by K. Brown, *Wall Street Journal*, 1 October 1997. Those of us over 65 are generally unable to contract with providers for services outside the umbrella of Medicare regulation and approval. A provider who would agree to see us privately must forego the treatment of all Medicare patients for two years.

3. A corollary of this illusion is faith in the utility of regulations. See, for example, the feature article by P. Alper, MD in the *Wall Street Journal*, 5 November 1997. In an effort to contain costs and combat fraud, regulations have become so complex and onerous that every possible action appears to be either forbidden or compulsory. Even this might not be too terrible, except that there is so much ambiguity that it is often not possible to tell which is which.

4. The definition has become increasingly procrustean. R. Morgan, MD, and associates, "The Medicare–HMO Revolving Door," *New England Journal of Medicine*,

17 July 1997, point out that there is an increasingly stringent selection bias in HMO enrollment and exit.

5. We are now beginning to see an ominous turn in medical teaching. Increasingly the curriculum is under pressure to conform to the assumptions of government regulation or corporate policy. See, for example, an article by L. Barness, MD in the *New England Journal of Medicine*, 31 July 1997.

6. Fortunately, a strategy of impeding information in the service of corporate policy is ultimately a losing game. See E. Ginsberg and M. Ostow, *New England Journal of Medicine*, 3 April 1997. Their view is that the managed care model will not remain stable because the law of diminishing returns will apply to further cost savings, and lack of suitable redress for undertreatment will create increasing dissatisfaction.

7. Autonomy and the regulatory mind are, of course, polar opposites. See editor J. Kassirer, MD, *New England Journal of Medicine*, 1 July 1997. He warns against the hazards of micromanagement of medical practice by means of legislation.

*Chapter 6*

# What Healthcare Professionals Want

### I'm a Doctor, Not a Paper Pusher
by Jody Robinson

Starting this July, under the federal government's new Medicare Correct Coding Policy, doctors will be spending a lot more time on paperwork rather than patient care. In fact, documentation requirements are on the verge of subsuming medical care itself. These regulations started as a legitimate effort to determine that services government pays for have actually been delivered. But they've developed into a Rube Goldberg system in which auditors with little or no medical training will determine if doctors are actually doing their jobs instead of committing fraud all day long.

Under little-publicized provisions of the 1996 Health Insurance Portability and Accountability Act (the Kennedy–Kassenbaum law), enforcement responsibility will rest with 450 FBI agents hired specifically for this purpose. This also means that if you are a Medicare patient, the FBI will have unfettered access to your medical records.

The new regulations, issued by the Health Care Financing Administration, are so heavy-handed that it is clear they have little or nothing to do with the care of the patient. For example, to justify a 25-minute visit with a Medicare patient, a physician will have to generate a written record including—just try to follow this—the chief complaint; an extended history of the present illness (four or more elements, or the status of, at least three chronic or inactive conditions); a review of systems (an inventory of two to nine bodily systems); pertinent past medical, family and social history; plus either a detailed examination (including at least six organ systems or body areas with at least two elements each or at least 12 elements in two or more organ systems or body areas), as well as two out of three either multiple diagnoses or management options, a moderate amount or complexity of data to be reviewed, along with the risk of complications or morbidity or mortality.

There's more. Somewhere along the line, a numbingly complex matrix of required elements must be consulted for each medical interaction to determine which level of office-visit service should be coded for billing to Medicare. Failure to do so with consistent accuracy can subject the miscreant physician to fines of up to $10,000 an incident. So the physician must turn to elaborate tables of symptoms and body parts to be sure that the reported number of findings are distributed among the right number of body systems and duly recorded.

The effective date of these new regulations was delayed to July from January after a howl of protest from physicians. But there is little indication that they will be substantially modified. They should be dumped altogether.

The concept of standardizing the work to be expected with various levels of care seems reasonable at first glance. Medical records, after all, once consisted of little more than scanty scribbled observations. But the days of undocumented medical treatment have long since passed. Physicians, who have labored for at least 30 years under the threat of malpractice litigation, long ago became conscientious at recording the details of significant findings and treatments.

A look at the new regulations leads to the unavoidable conclusion that a disproportionate amount of time will be consumed by pedantic record keeping, at the expense of the patient. The information mandated is so voluminous—lots of chaff for little or no wheat—that it's of no use to the next person to use the medical record either.

Such a single-minded focus on documentation may satisfy the bureaucrat and the accountant, but it can be hazardous to the patient. After all, a doctor can do only so much in 15 to 30 minutes. Every unnecessary or arbitrary documentation mandate takes away from the time available to evaluate systems, formulate a diagnosis or a treatment plan, explain the problem or write prescriptions . . . and, oh yes, comfort and console the patient. These requirements are demeaning to physicians, surely among the most skilled, educated and ethical professionals in our society.

The real purpose of these regulations is to find ways to reduce the payment for services provided to patients by applying the rule: *If it isn't documented, it didn't happen.*

How can a doctor keep the patient's needs foremost in mind when every interaction is laden with administrative burden and fraught with legal peril? "The secret of caring for the patient is to care for the patient," said the great early-20th-century physician Francis Peabody [corrected from the original]. To put it in our contemporary lingo, it's the patient, not the chart. Documentation should not become the tail that wags the dog.

On the other hand, if this is good medicine for doctors, perhaps every government official and employee should be subject to similar work-substantiation requirements. It might be instructive to have each of our public servants report minute-to-minute activities and accomplishments in comparable detail, so we could all know just where our tax dollars are going.[1]

## INTRODUCTION

The tent that covers the health professions is large indeed. There are physicians and nurses, psychologists and dentists, technicians, therapists, and specialists of every kind. All of them want the same things, such as productive work, authority congruent with responsibility, the respect of peers and colleagues, a working environment characterized by calmness and dignity, and compensation. Although this chapter is developed from the perspective of the physician, the same concerns apply to the extended family of healthcare disciplines and specialties.

Since the time of Aristotle, it has been known that productive work is one of the pillars of human happiness and fulfillment. At a minimum, this means that one can go home at the end of the day with the assurance that one's family is a bit more secure and that the world may be a slightly better place because of one's labor. Yet one does not live by productive work alone. There is also responsibility and authority. Balance between them is important. When they are not proportionate, demoralization and resentment are the likely consequences. Excessive responsibility without the authority to make necessary changes invites burnout. Authority without responsibility invites erratic judgment and the loss of respect of peers and subordinates.

Productive work also requires a bedrock of mutual respect from colleagues and peers. Nowhere is this point more applicable than in healthcare. The essence of professionalism is the exercise of independent judgment that builds from empirical data. For such judgment to be effective, the choices must be reasonable and congruent with the practice of other professionals with similar training and responsibility. To practice in isolation is to risk cumulative error and deviance from accepted parameters. To practice in an atmosphere in which sanctions have their source outside of a profession is to make the avoidance of risk the primary purpose of behavior. Such sanctions bias one's professional judgments toward decisions that are routine and restrict one's thinking to the path always traveled. But at times, the best professional judgments need to depart from the usual.

There is also the issue of calmness and dignity. Hospitals and clinics need to be orderly places, where rules are followed, where decorum is observed, and where professionals can work effectively. Ideally, the work environment is free from arbitrary political and administrative interference in clinical decisions and from excessive emotion. Ideally, it is a place where scientific decision making is supported and one person is in charge of the case, not a group with diluted responsibility.

There is also the matter of the amount of money that professionals should be paid. In general, professionals have a tendency to estimate the compensation they deserve by comparing themselves with friends that have similar backgrounds, education, and responsibilities. They compare the difficulty of their tasks with those of others in similar fields and they look for equity.

They consider the cost of education and other start-up expenses. They consider the hours that they spend at work and in self-education outside of work. In most instances, they believe that whatever compensation others in their profession have enjoyed in the past should be the baseline from which compensation should be projected.

Ideally, the free market should specify the value of medical care, just as it does for many goods and services. This ideal is distorted by a variety of factors such as long and expensive apprenticeships, political and corporate intrusiveness and constraints, unending and confusing national attitudes about the priorities of healthcare, and inequalities in the availability of funds to pay for care. It makes no sense to compensate a physician inadequately who cares for the poor while excessively compensating one who cares for the wealthy. Economic factors are not the only ones that require attention, however. For example, there is a natural human tendency to overvalue one's contributions when compared to those of others. Thus, some self-correcting mechanism needs to be found. Despite its limitations, there seems to be no better general model than the free market, and it is perhaps there that our efforts ought to be directed if we wish to introduce equity and responsibility into the compensation picture.[2]

## WHO ARE THESE PROFESSIONALS, ANYWAY?

A profession is more than a job. It is defined by a combination of attributes that imply independence of judgment and a high degree of individual personal responsibility. Professionals may expect to be treated with some deference when their expertise is grounded in a body of knowledge that is not widely held by the public. This knowledge does not consist of mere opinion, nor is it a collection of hunches or folklore. It is a coherent set of facts and inferences to which professionals subscribe. Although there may be differences of opinion at the edges, there remains, nevertheless, a core of facts and inferences that enjoy general agreement and that may be verified by those outside of the profession.

Professionals are charged with fiduciary responsibility for their clients. That is, the proper practice of the profession implies placement of the interests of the client before the income and convenience of the practitioner. Unless a legal principle is at issue, attorneys are constrained from advancing lawsuits that are likely to be more costly than they are worth. Teachers may not properly instruct students in fallacious ways, even if students desire it. Physicians may not properly treat nonexistent diseases or disorders, even if patients insist. Engineers may not properly use inferior designs or inadequate materials, even if their clients suggest it.

Fiduciary responsibility implies that professionals must be governed by ethical standards that surpass those that often prevail in the marketplace. This is a time-honored concept on which the majority of professionals agree.

Yet it conflicts with much of the prevailing ideology of the day because it suggests that some people take more responsibility than others. Enthusiastic egalitarians sometimes take exception to this ethical view and replace it with the notion that the prevailing standard should be whether an action is legal rather than whether it is proper. There is no easy resolution to this issue. Laws apply to everyone. Yet laws and the interpretation that individuals give to them change, and ethical standards may veer in different directions. For example, this is the case with rules that punish physicians who develop contracts with patients receiving Medicare for providing healthcare beyond that which the government approves.

Let us digress a moment and look at some of the Medicare rules in detail. As the federal law now stands, participation in Medicare Part A—the part that pays for hospital care—is mandatory if one receives Social Security benefits. This means that many Americans automatically become subject to Medicare regulations whether or not they wish to participate. In addition, the federal government enrolls all seniors in Medicare Part B (the part that pays for doctors' visits) unless patients choose not to join. If this were all there is to the rules, there would be little to be concerned about. However, beginning on January 1, 1998, a new Medicare Part B coercive rule was put into effect for persons over 65 years of age. Coercion occurs because the Federal Budget Act, which was enacted in 1997, contains a provision requiring any doctor who contracts for extra services with a Medicare patient to refrain from treating Medicare patients for two years. Because most physicians are unlikely to forgo their Medicare patients, this rule translates as follows: persons over 65 will have to join Medicare Part B if they want to see the doctor of their choice. Such patients may receive only such care as the Medicare bureaucracy approves.

One may view the preceding rule in several ways, but clearly, it amounts to the government twisting the arms of many elderly in ways to which they object. Moreover, the rule is a form of government intrusion that conflicts with patients exercising free choice. It does not take account of individuals who require greater amounts of care. Nor is it likely to improve the quality of care. Payments are capped for the time physicians spend treating individuals in Medicare Part B and the cap is barely sufficient to cover office expenses and minimal compensation. Because, like most people, physicians try to avoid living on the financial brink, they are likely to minimize the time they spend with Part B patients.

Authority arising from knowledge and fiduciary responsibility have no meaning if the profession loses control of the certification of its members. For example, if an institution conferred engineering credentials on its students without the expected training, it would be asserting that knowledge itself has no objective standard. Institutions, and even governments, have tried such experiments, and with predictable results. Similarly, if a government asserted that it alone could judge what is proper in a fiduciary relationship, the results would likely include the refusal of physicians to treat certain types of patients and declining standards of quality.

Self-governance is the defining feature of true professionalism. Without it, other attributes can easily be compromised. It is crucial to decide the qualifications for entry into the profession, to determine what standards must be upheld in order to remain a member of the profession, and to specify what the rules of membership in a profession shall be. Self-governance and accountability go hand in hand. Said differently, the goals of self-governance within a profession are to defend the capacity of professionals to make fact-based decisions and to avoid the erosions of this capacity that can often occur when there are political or corporate intrusions.

It is no secret that self-governance by professions has proved to be far from perfect, and the healthcare professions are not exceptions. A percentage of physicians engage in unethical (and often illegal) practices, including prescribing excessive amounts of addicting drugs, engaging in unnecessary operations, and recommending treatments for which there is no empirical foundation. It is for such reasons that government has felt it necessary to regulate professional practice by means of licensing boards that have the power to grant, withhold, or rescind the right to practice.

It is difficult to fault the government for wanting to develop such boards. Citizens need to be protected from those physicians who can do more harm than good. Moreover, left to themselves, professions might be tempted to abuse their autonomy by promoting self-aggrandizing policies at the expense of clients and society. Thus, a balance is necessary so that government may broadly regulate professional activity without interference in the ethical basis on which a profession's work depends. Granting these points, it is still necessary to point out that government is not wholly successful in its efforts to contain and direct professions. The number of medical licenses that are rescinded each year, the frequency with which physicians are placed on probationary status, and the high degree of medical fraud are signs that attempts to contain and direct professions are far from satisfactory.

If both professional self-governance and governmental regulation are imperfect, what alternatives are there? This question is answered in later chapters when we address the structure and function of organizations.

## PROFESSIONALS WANT DECISION AUTONOMY

Professional activity is the exercise of judgment. Although there are features of craftsmanship in many professional activities, the essential core of any profession is the exercise of independent assessment of problems and the proposal of solutions for which the practitioner is personally responsible. By necessity, professionals must live in a world of facts rather than wishes. They cannot blame society if their calculations are shown to be in error. They cannot plead that they were having a bad day or that their brain was impaired by the ingestion of too many Twinkies. If the bridges they design fall down, they are responsible, even if they were abused as children. This is what it means to be a professional.

Self-governance is not always the easiest of tasks. Telling the truth when everyone would rather embrace a preferred lie can be hazardous. For example, ineffective treatments might be cheaper than effective ones, and thus in the short run, profits might be maximized. Because cash flow is easily measured, while clinical effectiveness may take a long time to be shown, the honest scientific clinician may have to fight an up-hill battle. To speak the truth is to be willing to put your job on the line. Not to speak the truth is to cease to be a professional.

By accepting this degree of rigor for themselves, professionals expect that they will enjoy a degree of respect commensurate with their responsibilities and the risks they take. In a world that often favors the avoidance of accountability, professionals seldom have a choice other than accepting the world as it is. This situation not only requires that they refuse to accede to demands to compromise their judgment, but also that professionals may have to change jobs frequently because the world does not always respect their need for autonomy. It also means that professionals who are employed by large corporations or government, where those in charge are not accustomed to being told things they do not wish to hear, enter a world in which they may be unable to live up to the ethical standards of their profession.

Humans are social and hierarchical beings, and for many individuals who work in hierarchies, their goal is to rise to the top. This goal is not always fostered by adherence to observation and logic, however. Still, for the world to work, someone has to tell the truth. This is the niche properly inhabited by professionals. A practical consequence of this point is that professionals must be the leaders in the critical examination of their assumptions and working evidence in the light of newly discovered facts. Requirements for continuing education are one of the variables that distinguish the professional from many less information-rich activities of commerce or politics. Frequent consultation with colleagues is another variable. Unending self-education is a third.

The essential feature of continuing education, consultation, and self-education is that decisions should rest on a firm foundation of fact as derived from the best available research when combined with a critical eye for the use of logic. This means that those offering courses for professionals need to be scrutinized carefully for their motivation as well as their credentials. For example, a course for physicians which is designed by pharmaceutical companies must be evaluated carefully to assure that it is not just a forum for promoting the questionable use of a new and expensive drug. Likewise, an offering designed and funded by a company providing medical insurance should be examined for possible biases concerning the cost of diagnosis and treatment rather than therapeutic effectiveness.

To return to the point that someone needs to tell the truth, in recent years an academic fad has developed that explicitly denies the existence of objective truth. Derived from the work of the French philosopher Michel Foucault, the notion is that there are no truths and no facts. Rather, there is only political power. In Foucault's mind, the pursuit of truth is some type of sham that the powerful use to enhance their hegemony over those less powerful. One is tempted to dismiss this folly as beneath the threshold of useful discourse. Yet Foucault's so-called ideas have managed to ensconce themselves in many prestigious university settings. It is not sufficient simply to observe that Foucault's views were asserted without proof and thus expect them to disappear. Would that it were so. Rather, it is now necessary to restate repeatedly with clarity and conviction what was once commonly known: *some ideas are better than others.* The discourse on truth does not stop here. Critics often counter with statements like, "No idea is perfect." We agree, with the caveat that it is also true that over time those ideas that conform to observation and logic will prove to be the most useful because they are able to make progressively closer approximations to the truth.

Professionals must be among the leaders in the design of systems for the evaluation of quality. Without professional involvement, managers and clerks will assume the task of defining how a system should operate. Their frequent lack of understanding of the ideas and evidence from which a profession builds makes this solution hazardous. This means building systems of self-evaluation and stringent criteria of correction.

## WHAT IS SPECIFIC TO HEALTHCARE?

Nurses and physicians form the core of the healthcare professional team. They are assisted by a spectrum of other members that includes therapists and technicians from many specialties. The team is united by a set of assumptions that often are not seen in other areas of employment, namely that the team assumes responsibility for the patient for an indefinite future. Once treatment begins, it can not be abandoned for as long as the situation requires. Resignation from cases is possible under certain circumstances, but when it occurs arrangements must be made for continuity of care at the level of intensity and thoroughness which the situation demands.

There is also the need for division of responsibility and the maintenance of clear boundaries between professions. Patients have the right to expect that jurisdictional disputes will be kept to a minimum and that they will not compromise care. They have the right to expect a coherent treatment plan that integrates the work of all the disciplines into an efficient and cost-effective whole. Unfortunately, some mistakes will occur. When they do, the best chance for rectification is if they occur in a context of responsibility and thoroughness.

## THE WESTERN MEDICAL TRADITION

The ideals on which Western medicine builds follow the tradition of the civilization that had its origin in Athens over 2,400 years ago. Pericles expressed these ideals with clarity in his funeral oration for the Athenian soldiers killed in the war with Sparta. There are three basic ideas: that the individual is important, that democracy is the proper form of government, and that happiness depends on freedom, which in turn depends on courage. Central to Pericles's message is the concept that there is a necessary and insoluble bond between freedom and responsibility.

If the Periclean model is taken as the ideal for the relationship between the individual and government, so another model of the same period in Greece remains the ideal of the practice of medicine. This is the Hippocratic ideal. In the physician's oath attributed to Hippocrates, three salient commandments are visible: that the physician's authority derives from his virtue as an honorable agent of the patient, that a physician–patient fiduciary responsibility exists, and that the profession is responsible to itself for the development of the standards by which practice is conducted.[3]

Seldom are noble ideals fully achieved, and those that apply to medicine are not exceptions. Hippocrates gave us what perhaps remains the best single statement of the practice of medicine. Do physicians live up to these expectations? The answer is, "Some of the time, but not always." Why only some of the time? Part of the answer is that over the last five decades another model has developed to compete with the original requirements of Hippocrates—the contract model.

While the Hippocratic tradition and its ethical correlates served patients well for centuries, conflicting traditions in this century have brought its relevance into question. For example, some have criticized the assumption embedded in the Hippocratic tradition that the physician knows best. Another criticism is that physicians assume the right to use the power of their office in a paternalistic manner. These concerns are not without merit and they in part reflect the changing attitudes towards religion in the West. Until early in this century, there was a quasi-religious aspect to medical treatment. The physician was seen as an instrument of divine intervention, which inevitably fostered the development of paternalistic attitudes. Individual autonomy was compromised by the general attitude that patients ought properly to obey physicians' orders and that they should passively accept the idea that they would receive treatment and information only to the extent that these were in their best interest.

The contract model has its origins in the idea of individual empowerment. This model states that the relationship between physicians and patients is one of equality, requiring free disclosure of all relevant information and treatment options. Said another way, physicians and nurses are essentially technical functionaries who contract to "patch up" individuals in return for money. This view avoids the pitfalls of paternalism. Further, in its ideal form, it maximizes the dignity and humanity of each patient. When illness or injury is curable, most of us would prefer it.

Yet there are times when the contract model is less comforting. When we must confront a lingering fatal illness or one that promises only greater pain and disability each day, then paternalism may be what we want. Hippocrates, or his deputy, will keep the secrets when, in his or her judgment, they should be kept, and when keeping them gives us a bit of hope and comfort. The contract model is not congenial to this form of charity, while the Hippo-cratic model assumes that charity is offered and accepted in certain circum-stances. Medical care at the end of the twentieth century in the United States turns out to be a cloudy mixture of these two models. Moreover, much of our confusion about and dissatisfaction with our healthcare system comes about when the provider is in one model while the patient is in the other.

## THE VETERINARY MODEL

Although the two models described above, living in uneasy compromise with each other, make up the dominant style of healthcare in America, there is another way of looking at the problem, one that is seen more frequently in countries that embrace the concept of the welfare state. This might be called the Veterinary model, in which healthcare is conferred upon the peo-ple without regard to their wishes or their consent. The government knows best, in this view, and people can't be expected to be able to understand enough to see that it is all done for their own good. All healthcare is or-ganized around public health models, as if the needs of everyone were iden-tical. There may be immunizations and pure water in the public supply, but there will be little consultation with the recipients of care—what do they know anyway?

The Veterinary model thus contains the worst features of the Hippocratic and the contract models. There is no place for charity and emotional com-fort, nor is there any place for personal choice and autonomy. There is the implicit assumption that the state owns your body and will enhance health or dispose of you as it sees fit—but always, of course, with the idea that the primary value is the "public good." The Veterinary model promises equality of care, nothing else. And the promise of equality is a powerful attractor of political support. Perhaps it will not be too lacking in charity to observe, however, that where it is most vigorously advocated, there is generally a privileged political class with access to alternative means of treatment.

But which model of care do healthcare professionals prefer? Like all the rest of humanity, there are advocates of each model, or compromises among them, at every level of the healthcare professions. A pluralistic society allows for a place for each, whether it is the public health officer, the pediatrician, or the surgeon. Many perspectives may be seen. The professional schools, the government, and the third-party payers each have some influence on the selection of those who enter the professions, and thus the future may be shaped by these choices.

## WHAT ABOUT RIGHTS?

Human rights are an obligatory topic when discussing any healthcare system. As noted, rights concerning medical care are usually more in the realm of political slogans than meaningful concepts. "Rights advocates" assert the right to treatment, the right to avoid treatment, the right to alternative treatment, and even the right to die as if these were compatible and mutually commensurate concepts. They are not. The right to die provides a convenient example.

In recent years an idea has developed that there exists a "right to die" and that, therefore, there must exist a complementary obligation for physicians to assist patients in exercising this right. When the idea is discussed, there are always the pious reassurances that strict controls ought to be observed: the patient must have a terminal illness, the patient must be of sound mind, and the patient must have intolerable and untreatable pain. Given these strict controls, it is argued that physicians have the obligation to provide a guaranteed death should the patient so request.

Most healthcare professionals are not so sure. Each of the controls associated with the right to die idea seems to be far too elastic, thus in principle making euthanasia suitable for a large range of individuals for whom it was not intended. For example, from one perspective, we all have a terminal illness, although for most of us it has yet to be identified. In addition, even with tightly defined criteria applying to terminally ill diagnoses and prognoses, our capacity to say when "terminality" begins is a matter of conjecture. Similarly, how is the soundness of mind to be determined and who is to determine it? Finally, at what point does pain become intolerable, and who decides whether all plausible methods of amelioration have been exhausted?

Vigorous assertion of what is now sometimes called the "right to assisted suicide" may lead to legal permissiveness. Should this happen, the concept could quickly develop its own momentum—that is, once it is legal it may perhaps be recommended. If it becomes legal, a family may perhaps, implicitly or explicitly, encourage or even coerce the decision to initiate an assisted suicide. It is because of possible coercion that most healthcare professionals express a deeply felt skepticism of this newly discovered "right." Except for the occasional zealot, they recognize how fallible they can be and that ideas and criteria change. They wish, rightly, to avoid having to decide who is terminally ill, who is of sound mind, and who is intolerable pain.[4]

Healthcare professionals usually have a clearer idea than others that rights come with responsibilities, since the "rights" of the recipients imply the obligation of the donors to provide whatever these goods are presumed to be. As we noted, "entitlement" is a more precise term. But entitlements become an unstable concept as the expectations of the donors and recipients must necessarily diverge on the questions of quantity and quality.

## HEALTHCARE PROFESSIONALS AND MEDICAL QUALITY

Patients have different standards for judging the quality of treatment depending on their particular circumstances. Seldom is this the perspective of physicians. For them, quality is getting the correct diagnosis as quickly and efficiently as possible and applying a treatment that is known to be effective on the basis of well-designed and scientifically valid studies. Oddly, this quest for accurate diagnosis is a preoccupation of professionals, yet patients, insurance companies, and regulatory bodies often do not share it. Patients are generally happy to remain in the mode of accepting the authority of the physician, at least in the matter of diagnosis and treatment. On the other hand, insurance companies often seem skeptical about the idea that precise diagnosis is necessary. Precise diagnosis may require excessive laboratory tests. Insurance companies, therefore, tend to frown on what they see as indulging the physician's curiosity. There is a catch here, however: if a diagnosis is in error, it is the liability of the physician, not the insurance company.

Government and regulatory authorities also often have only casual interest in diagnostic accuracy. Their perspective is predictability and consistency of diagnosis and close correspondence between diagnosis and treatment. This perspective is derived from two of their primary tasks, statistical reporting and fraud reduction. Rare diagnoses, even if correct, do not serve these purposes well. And nothing is more distressing to the statistically minded bureaucrat than to find that a physician has used a nonstandard or innovative treatment for a common illness, even if such treatment is clearly indicated as a necessary departure in the service of individualized care.

Precision in diagnosis and skill in carrying out the indicated treatment are not the whole story in quality assessment. Earlier we noted that it is not logically possible to maximize the three competing healthcare variables of quality, availability, and cost. Rather, it is the task of professionals to achieve the most effective compromise among these variables. A simple fact of clinical life is the following: it is often necessary to design treatments on an individualized basis. For one patient or one condition, precision may be most important. In other cases, timeliness becomes the most salient concern. Cost must always be considered, but some will find it less compelling than will others.[5]

## WHAT ABOUT ALTERNATIVE TREATMENTS?

Enter the issue of "alternative" treatments and their place in a comprehensive healthcare perspective. There are so many concepts and procedures that claim a place in this domain that it is not possible to consider all of them. Ancient and modern ideas coexist, from Egyptian, Vedic, and Chinese medical writing to modern inventions of crystal power and "therapeutic touch." Some treatments have more plausibility than others, and all share at least a measure of attractiveness that gathers some adherents.

One common feature unites these treatments. They have not been shown to be effective or valid by well-designed clinical trials using the tools of observation and logic and such experimental methods as random assignment of treatment groups and blind assessment of the hoped-for therapeutic results. Practitioners of the alternatives depend on the faith and enthusiasm of their patients and on the unsupported authority of their teachers. When pressed for evidence of effectiveness, alternative practitioners point to testimonials and anecdotes. Critical thinking is seldom valued. Skepticism is turned aside by the claim that critics lack open-mindedness.

Is mainstream medicine so different? In many ways, the answer is no. Many of the concepts and procedures that are part of mainstream medical care have not been subjected to sufficiently rigorous testing. In their efforts to relieve distress, and when their scientific training is exhausted, physicians are apt to search in such dusty bins of knowledge as grandmother's tales of miraculous cures. An unfortunate fact of clinical life is that there are many important things that are not fully understood. When a clinical problem emerges that is beyond the light of currently understood science, physicians do the best they can with hunches and hopes. To do less is to ignore the humanity of those patients who desire to hold on to hope when science can not provide comfort.

There are, however, important distinctions here, and they have to do with the method of acquiring knowledge. For the scientific practitioner, knowledge has greater value as it receives accumulating support from empirical testing. Given two diagnostic formulations or two possible treatments, the superior idea is the one that is more supportable scientifically. Unsupportable treatments are gradually abandoned. To be sure, this process takes time, and there are periods in which concepts that will turn out to be superior and inferior coexist. However, eventually, good diagnosis and treatment forces out the bad. Those treatments that are embraced as "alternative" often fail this test.

The role of the genuine healthcare professional is thus in part one of a scientific practitioner and educator. Professionals recognize a duty to state clearly that some practices are superior to others. They must be willing to say that some concepts are incorrect no matter how many others believe in them or wish they would be true. Because of this approach, the true professional may be criticized as intolerant or "elitist" for insisting that some ideas are better than other ideas. To recognize the duty to make such distinctions, however, is the very definition of a professional.

## AN EQUITABLE LEGAL ENVIRONMENT

Human agencies can be organized in two general ways. The ancient method is to encase behaviors in a web of authority and rules. The more modern and generally more effective method is to construct incentives that will move human actions in the desired direction. Rules tend to solidify existing practice, while systems of incentive allow for adaptation and evolution. Behavior is shaped towards optimization by allowing each member of the system to use his or her wits to accomplish goals rather than scheming to circumvent the rules.

Every system needs rules but, as we have stressed, these ought to be minimized as much as possible if only because rules tend to foster deviant behavior rather than the hoped-for progress. Further, we have also stressed that most rules work best if they are derived from within the profession rather than imposed by external forces. These views seldom mesh with reality, however. For example, at this moment in time, it is not thought odd that attorneys form a significant presence on boards governing the practice of physicians, engineers, or any other profession. (It would be thought odd indeed for governing committees of attorneys to be staffed by non-attorneys.) The fact that attorneys are present on non-attorney boards has its own logic. Boards need to understand the law. But law and professional ethics often conflict. Sometimes they do so in instances where the ethical principles receive public support while the law forbids or constrains. Healthcare designed to fit the individual is perhaps the most obvious example of this point.

Another area of law and regulation that requires urgent attention is the current practice of tort litigation as it applies to professional liability. It is simply not reasonable to assert, as trial lawyers do, that if something bad happens, it must necessarily be someone else's fault. Nor is it reasonable to assert that the way to identify the bearer of liability is to find the person or institution that has the most money, however distant their association with the injury. Medical practice could be far better, far more efficient, and far more equitable if the law could recognize that bad results sometimes come from genuine negligence, while at other times these unfortunate results stem from uncontrollable factors. Genuine negligence requires just compensation. Uncontrollable factors require another response.

Sometimes a calamity evolves slowly and thus evades our normal alarm mechanisms. This is the case with the current system of torts and liabilities primarily because the tort liability system has yet to come under the control of any natural means of market regulation. Two features of the system prevent market discipline from restoring fiscal sense. The first is our custom that the cause for litigation is limited only by the attorney's imagination regardless of cost or benefit. The second is the custom of contingency fees.

Legal principles of other nations have recognized the inherent conflict of interest in contingency fees, and so their use is restricted or forbidden. In the United States, the justification has been that such a fee mechanism gives the poor a ready access to jurisprudence. In times past, it was the custom that the client would elect to pay the attorney directly or ask him to accept a contingency fee. Now the choice is the attorney's, and most ask for a lucrative percentage of the final award. On this point, there is an occasional ray of hope. Recently, for example, a number of judges in the pending diet pill litigation have expressed their concern about the anticipated lawyers' fees in class action suits and have considered the alternative of trying each prospective case individually.

In the current environment of movement toward a standard of strict liability, a defense based on the absence of demonstrated fault holds little promise of being successful. Unlucky events may trigger a large award. Liability insurance is then seen as the source of compensation. This drive for strict liability and perfect compensation, undaunted by economic reality or the implications for quality healthcare, must eventually destroy its own source of sustenance, just as a parasite may kill its host and thus prevent its own survival. (As an aside, it is worth underscoring the fact that lawyers do not exercise the same peer review process over colleagues' day-to-day legal behavior as do physicians regarding their own behavior. Here, an inherent conflict between healthcare and law are readily apparent. Day-to-day peer review in medicine, which has the goal of improving quality of care, is in the best interests of both physicians and patients. Peer review in law, if it existed, might well seriously constrain the earning power of lawyers.)

What is to be done? First, we must recognize the ultimate implications of a system of unconstrained tort liability. It is a juggernaut that by its internal logic must relentlessly grow until it is constrained by economic decline of the supporting society. Second, we must realize that economic consequences must be considered as part of any system of compensation. For example, some obstetricians have been forced out of practice by insurance premiums that may exceed their incomes. Their work might then fall to midwives, whose insurance premiums can then begin to escalate without natural bounds.

If we should not continue the unlimited subsidy of trial lawyers, how can we preserve the access to all of fair compensation? One alternative easily comes to mind. It is borrowed from current policies to provide medical care for the poor. Attorneys in liability cases could be paid by a state agency set up for this purpose and modeled on Medicare and Medicaid. Attorneys could receive the same hourly rate that physicians are paid for treating patients. This would not only assure the representation of clients with meritorious claims, but it would also guarantee fair professional compensation. It would also assure that injured parties receive the full amount of the award. Most important, it would diminish the incentive to file frivolous claims.

## PROFESSIONALS WANT GOOD COMPENSATION

As a rule, professionals are not egalitarians, at least insofar as compensation is concerned. They want to be paid above the average. They justify this view on the basis that there are many contributions they have given to society that are not easily accounted for. Their education and training are, in general, longer than that of nonprofessionals, and there are both direct and opportunity costs that are the consequences of such training. They also note that as a group professionals have burdens of hands-on responsibility for the lives and safety of others. Because in the last analysis they are selling judgment, they expect to be paid well when the judgment is good. On the other hand, they expect sanctions if their judgments are bad.

Healthcare professionals, and especially physicians, at least in the past 40 years, have had these expectations substantially fulfilled. Physicians' net income accounts for about 8% of the total national healthcare expenditure. The emergence of this compensation by indirect means has introduced some distortions into the process, however. For example, when the patient is not included in the loop and insurance companies set fees according to what to them seems reasonable, there is a bias toward measurable activity. This usually means that a physical procedure, such as surgery, is valued more highly than the apparently passive process of thinking, advising, and educating the patient. Recognizing this skewed set of incentives, physicians are attracted to specialties with a greater number of measurable procedures.

More than others, physicians are subject to a variety of measures, explicit and hidden, that amount to control of income by law or regulation. This often comes in the form of a decision by insurance companies or the government that they will reduce payments from previously paid amounts. Already mentioned Medicare rules prevent physicians from billing patients for the balance. As in any system of legal constraint on the free market, this can lead to shortages of more valued services. The market in medical care has hardly been free from constraint for a long time, however. Whenever there is a displacement in place or time between service and payment, distortions occur. When third-party mediators come into play, this distortion is amplified.

## CONCLUDING COMMENTS

Asking what healthcare professionals want invites a far more complex set of answers than at first might be anticipated. Moreover, the complexity continues because of the number of players in the healthcare arena. Government, insurance companies, HMOs, private practitioners, physicians groups, nurses groups, labor unions, diseases-oriented groups, and so forth—all are there and actively participating.

What then is the key point to be derived from this situation? We suggest the following: until there is clarification about the goals of our healthcare system, deciding what healthcare professionals want, and operationalizing our judgments simply will not happen.

## NOTES

1. Clearly, if physicians actually complied with these regulations, assuming that it is possible to do so, they would see fewer patients for shorter actual time and make less money—not counting the occasional $10,000 fines. Regulation which is this fatuous cannot be uniformly enforced. This makes us suspicious that the real intention is to provide bureaucrats with a club to beat professionals who displease them through selective enforcement. Reprinted with permission of the *Wall Street Journal* (April 1, 1998) (© 1999 Dow Jones & Company, Inc. All rights reserved) and the author, Dr. Jody Robinson, who practices internal medicine in Washington, D.C.

2. D. Armey, majority leader of the US House of Representatives, *Wall Street Journal*, 17 November 1998, discusses the perverse incentives that may arise from a payment system based on the government as the single payer. He advocates the expansion of plans based on medical savings accounts.

3. For sardonic amusement, see A. Pruchnicki, *New England Journal of Medicine*, 27 November 1997, in which he imagines Hippocrates at an employment interview with a modern HMO.

4. Paul McHugh, writing in the *American Scholar*, Winter, 1997, discusses the problem of physician-assisted suicide by analyzing the phenomenon of Dr. Kevorkian.

5. Allocation of clinical resources makes it necessary to have a clear position on rationing. D. Asch and P. Ubel, *New England Journal of Medicine*, 5 June 1997, discuss the problem of rational clinical choices that take cost into account. Their point is that judgments of this type are not properly considered as rationing, but that compromises must necessarily be made.

*Chapter 7*

# What Healthcare Payers Want

## INTRODUCTION

The people are the payers. Whether out-of-pocket or through insurance premiums or taxes, the great majority of Americans pay the costs of healthcare. A long-standing and well-entrenched distortion has led many citizens to believe that the payers are insurance carriers and the government. Consequently, effective solutions to our healthcare difficulties have become harder. Why? On balance, the introduction of a third party, such as an insurance company, tends to decrease efficiency and, in turn, increase cost.

Nevertheless, third-party payers have emerged over the past 40 years for understandable reasons. To their credit, they have brought improvement in some areas of healthcare utilization and access. In addition, through advertising and other means, such as providing healthcare options to businesses, they have made the benefits of modern medicine known to a large percentage of the US population. Because paying taxes or insurance premiums amounts to prepaying for one's healthcare, patients have had an incentive to seek medical interventions earlier than might otherwise have occurred. Still, when the balance sheet is evaluated, not only have third-party payers been a major contributor to both the increased costs of healthcare and patient dissatisfaction, but it is also rare that anyone claims they have improved the quality of care.

## THIRD-PARTY PAYERS—THE HISTORY

What, then, is the history of this reliance on third-party payers? Given their history, why do third-party payers have such a stranglehold on healthcare in the United States? What are the implications of continuing third-party payments for the future? The events associated with World War II have been mentioned. Employers faced serious difficulties in their efforts to recruit skilled labor due to price and wage controls. A natural tendency for employers was to look for fringe benefits that would make their jobs more attractive while avoiding entanglements in a web of regulations. Because at the time the cost of healthcare was relatively small, employers could offer healthcare coverage without a major investment of resources.

In addition to relatively lower costs, the decade of the 1940s was one in which the expectations for medical care were not so large as they are now. Adults of that time were accustomed to a different type of medicine. Siblings died in childhood. Polio, rheumatic fever, whooping cough, diphtheria, scarlet fever, "lockjaw," St. Vitus dance, and many other life-threatening diseases were commonly discussed and frequent visitors to the average family. Physicians did what they could, which often was not much other than providing a measure of comfort and reassurance. Many children were born at home. Hospital stays were infrequent and often ominous in implication. Tuberculosis and schizophrenia were responsible for a large number of hospital admissions. Memorial Day was an opportunity for a family outing at the cemetery in a ritual of remembrance for those who had "passed away."

Participating in a war of epic proportions which affected literally every American, and with the future in doubt, health insurance seemed a welcome respite from one minor worry, that of paying the doctor's bill. An anecdote illustrates the feelings of the time. Recently one of the authors was having dinner with an old friend, a distinguished physician who had spent his professional career in the Public Health Service and who had received numerous awards. The friend was board certified in two medical specialties and several sub-specialties. He had held clinical, administrative, and teaching positions all over the world. At age 60, it seemed he would be a good observer of the trends of medical care costs and methods of payment. As the evening progressed, we came to the question of what it was like to be sick and without insurance in the 1940s. He described his own experience as a boy who developed appendicitis. The doctor came, made the diagnosis, and performed the necessary operation. His father paid the doctor by giving him his double-barreled shotgun. At the time, such transactions were not thought odd.

Times change, and since the 1940s there has been an ever increasing dependence on third-party coverage (no doubt, in part, because shotguns are an inconvenient medium of exchange). With these changes, there has emerged the illusion that third-parties, be they insurance companies or governmental entities, are the actual payers of healthcare and that medical care is (or should be) "free." Yet, as we have stressed repeatedly, once a valuable resource is perceived as free, it rapidly becomes a great deal more expensive because "free" resources inevitably spiral to overutilization. Applying this axiom to healthcare, it was inevitable that healthcare boundaries would expand. First, the effective treatments were covered by third parties. Second, patients began to insist that probably effective treatments should be covered. And so on. At the end of this exercise, it is common to find that many patients insist that any intervention which they believe might be helpful should be covered. Never mind that there is no evidence to suggest that many putative interventions work. Patients have paid in advance for the interventions they desire. Once this attitude dominates patients' thinking, they lose control of the contractual basis with providers and they abandon responsibility for contributing to a rational healthcare system. In turn, patients become increasingly dissatisfied, costs explode, and quality succumbs to increasingly frantic attempts of third parties to reestablish some sort of supply-demand equilibrium. Maybe the shotgun, or barter in general, has something to be said for it; at least the sanctity or the sanity of the contract between the provider and the consumer is preserved.

Patients are not entirely to blame for the current state of our healthcare system. Third parties are in no way immune from the cognitive distortions that envelop patients. Just as dislocation in time and space between service and payment contribute to patients' perceptions that care is free, so do the perceptions of third-party decision makers who begin to believe that care must be rationed to control overuse. The parallel illusion for the third-party executives is that they "own" the care, and that they must protect it from such overuse by law (in the case of government), or constraints and deception (in the case of private corporations). Worse still, at least in the case of government, they begin to believe and act as if they own the patients' bodies. Once these illusions are in place, perverse incentives enter the picture.

## THE VESTED INTERESTS OF THIRD PARTIES

Institutions have vested interests just as individuals do. As yet, however, these interests have failed to receive sufficient scrutiny. Whatever the institution in question, the people who work within it develop a group loyalty that is at once subtle and powerful. Such behavior is not unexpected. It is part of the evolutionary past that we bring to the present. As a species, we prefer to operate in small groups, to establish structure and hierarchies within our groups, and to defend our groups against other groups.

In the modern world, one of the groups to which people belong is found in the workplace. It is this congregation that earns part of our loyalty, largely because it is responsible for the allocation of resources received by group members. Leaders are often idealized, or at least given the provisional benefit of the doubt. Members expect to be treated fairly and generally seek to turn in a good day's work for a just day's pay. While members may not always enjoy the company of their co-workers, more often than not they develop a functional loyalty and defend even disliked members against criticism by outsiders. This loyalty is a powerful force, which is buoyed by considerable emotional capital. Organizations need to fail to reciprocate their members' loyalty repeatedly before members will abandon their emotional attachment to the group and seek membership elsewhere.

Given the above, it is not surprising that governments and corporations often develop idiosyncratic goals. Nor is it surprising that these goals are out of step with those of the larger society. For example, consider those employees of the Internal Revenue Service who seem to prefer to enhance the glory of the Service rather than to deal fairly and ethically with taxpayers. Rewards and sanctions, two of the key currencies of human behavior, are the usual culprits underlying such behavior. Groups survive in part because they promise that sacrifices and efforts will be rewarded with reciprocal donations, and it is part of human nature to work for the enhancement of groups in which we are valued members.

What may be said about the vested interests of insurance companies? This is not a hard call. Insurance companies, like all corporations, exist to generate profits for their shareholders and salaries and benefits for their employees. Other considerations are secondary. Executives who fail to embrace this concept may justly be called to account and subjected to discipline or termination. Employees whose efforts deviate from this goal are not likely to receive promotions. The goal is unambiguous: increase the cash flow and the profit by maximizing the input of revenue and decreasing the costs of operation.

In the case of healthcare insurance, the means to accomplish increased cash flow and maximized profits are relatively straightforward. Begin by offering a wide scope of treatments and procedures to be covered; then set premiums at the limits that the average customer will pay. When the limits of profitable treatments and procedures have been reached, the task becomes one of changing the rules such that the customers/patients no longer enjoy certain choices and decision-making autonomy. Once revenue has been maximized, the primary way to increase profit is to decrease costs by constructing institutional barriers to service delivery. New organizational forms are created with the purpose of restricting the demand for services. These new entities must be given appealing names in order to disguise their real purpose. "Health maintenance organizations" is a frequent choice. Yet, because insurance companies operate in a competitive environment, the increase-profit/reduce-costs objective must be disguised through creative advertising. It is also helpful for the goal of profit maximization if the legal and regulatory environment is congenial. Well-targeted political contributions often follow in efforts to lubricate progress towards this objective.[1]

## THE GOVERNMENT AS A THIRD-PARTY PAYER

Governments have vested interests as well. However, unlike corporations, they are burdened with an additional conflict of interest. The function of the corporation is to make money, while the government is charged with the task of acting in the best interest of the citizen. This injunction is not always congruent with the competing goal of increasing the size, budget, scope, and power of the civil servant's group—that is, the government agency or bureau to which an employee owes his or her loyalty. In effect, the government is under a continuing moral hazard that drives it toward behavior similar to the corporation. Put another way, government departments begin to look like insurance companies when they enter the healthcare arena.

None of this is to suggest that altruism is absent from the considerations of corporations or governments. Personnel in each generally wish to do what they perceive as the right thing, namely to invent and contribute to a healthcare system that offers good, inexpensive, and available healthcare. Still, good intentions are relentlessly eroded by a gradient of perverse incentives. When the showdown finally comes, the agents of government or insurance companies must, if they are to remain a respected group member, follow the interests of the group to which they owe the primary loyalty.

## THE LEGITIMATE CONCERNS OF THIRD-PARTY PAYERS

Healthcare in its fundamentals consists of transactions between patients and professionals who are skilled in the art and science of diagnosis and therapeutics. Payment mechanisms remain ancillary to this process. Yet in recent times the cart has come before the horse, with the essential concerns of healthcare being guided and even determined by payment methods. As this process has advanced, the percentage of the healthcare dollar allocated to overhead and administration has shown exponential growth, while that allocated to direct service (clinical care) has remained constant or even showed some decline. In today's complex world of corporate and government power, there is a real danger that this process may undergo a malignant transformation, with near-total absorption of the real service by an inadvertent alliance of administrators, regulators, and litigators.

That said, a realistic assessment indicates that various indirect payment schemes will be with us for a long time to come. It is therefore important to consider the institutional goals and concerns of insurance companies and government agencies. Some of these are reasonable and legitimate, while others are in need of being examined and reined in. The key place to start is with the structure of incentives. Perverse incentives must be nudged, and nudged significantly, in the direction of efficiency, productivity, and stability—that is, towards incentives that are acceptable to patients, providers, and payers. How this might be done is the topic of the next few chapters. However, this much seems clear. Whatever system might eventually emerge, there will be a need for some oversight and quality assurance by government as well as some financial risk sharing for catastrophic events by insurance companies.

What, then, are the proper concerns of government and insurance companies? Do they have any common interests? At one level, the answer is yes. When government or insurance company employees are sick, just like everyone else, they would much prefer access to solid, responsible, well-educated and well-trained professionals who know how to find out what is wrong and to do something effective about it. From this perspective, government and insurance carrier employees have an interest in a healthcare system that allows for high-quality diagnosis and treatment. Moreover, it is more pleasant as well as easier to work with a system that will produce a rational output for every unique input.

### Flexibility

From another perspective, insurance carriers have an interest in a healthcare system that is flexible enough to absorb innovative processes and techniques that become available because of scientific progress. At first, this idea may seem to be at odds with a fundamental bureaucratic tenet that innovation is to be avoided because it requires the upgrading of regulations. Yet the advantages of improved effectiveness benefit all. Still, in recent years it has become fashionable to attribute the rapid increase in medical care costs to precisely these technological innovations. As noted, it seems more reasonable that these improvements should reduce unit costs while increasing quality and availability. This has been the experience in most businesses. When technological advances fail to reduce costs and increase quality, the fault may not lie in the innovative process itself, but rather with the distorted system of incentives that third-party reimbursement schemes allow. For example, a reimbursement plan that is insensitive to costs will naturally foster new methods of diagnosis and treatment which share this perspective. On the other hand, a managed care environment that is sensitive only to costs and not to quality will not be congenial to any new techniques unless cost cutting is the main feature.

### Quality Providers

From yet another perspective, third-party payers have an interest in fostering a corps of professionals who are ethically sound, have excellent cognitive skills, and who are energetic in the pursuit of clinical knowledge. These professionals should be confident of their abilities and be comfortable with making independent judgments based on emerging clinical facts. They should be self-reliant, confident, honorable people whose first concern is the optimal care of the patient. In short, they should be the kind of people that administrators and managers would wish for as caretakers for members of their own families.

## Compromises

In an idealized world, third-party payers also want a reasonable balance of quality of care, equitable accessibility, and stable costs. These goals are laudable enough, although as noted, it is just not possible to maximize all three goals simultaneously. Just as engineers cannot make a machine equally good, cheap, and fast, so healthcare planners cannot make a system that is fully satisfactory in all aspects. Compromises need to be made. In the practical world where most of us spend most of our time, this means selecting the variable that is the least visible and ask it to bear the greatest burden of the compromise. Both the cost of healthcare and accessibility are unlikely candidates. Patients are generally sensitive to both; thus, there are constraints on the degree to which compromises of cost and accessibility are workable. Quality is another matter. What does and does not constitute quality healthcare is less clear to the average patient. Thus, quality frequently becomes the area in which compromises occur. Reducing quality invites its own problems, however, largely because professionals have a far better understanding of the concept of quality. Because they do, their sapiential authority now becomes a problem for managers and administrators. The fact/ value dichotomy again asserts itself. Managers begin to search for professionals whose sapietiality is less authoritative. They want professionals who are "team players," and who can be counted on to keep the interests of the institution firmly in mind—that is, people who will, when the chips are down, do what they are told to do.

## Effective Monitoring

The managers and administrators of third-party payers want effective monitoring of efficiency. They also want to be able to measure quality in absolute terms and to be sensitive to possible adverse trends. However, when it comes time to define the variables by which quality of care delivery is to be measured, perverse incentives again come to the fore. Even in the ideal world, there is an unavoidable tension between the precision and utility of measurements. One cannot simultaneously maximize both. The usual result is that the quality measures that are selected are strong on precision and weak on utility. If something is easy to measure, it is often easy to convince oneself that it has some relevance in the quest for quality. Once convinced, it is but a small step to the assumption that what can not be measured easily can safely be ignored. Given such reasoning, there is a natural human tendency to assume that the measures one is using are valid monitors of proper care. The selection of quality measures thus becomes critical for the well-being of the institution. (If later there are quibbles that the chosen measures are not fully adequate, the rejoinder quickly comes that it is important to continue their use anyway because, above all, comparable data must be collected in order to look for important secular trends.)

## Stability

Managers and administrators in corporations and government ideally want to have stability in their overhead and nondirect service costs. Control of costs is one of the hallmarks of the competent manager. Stockholders, directors, and senior civil servants are watchful to assure that waste is minimized and efficiency is promoted. It is for this reason that zero-based budgeting has become an increasingly popular management tool. Bonuses and incentive pay depend on prudent use of financial resources. Unfortunately, direct service costs are not always seen as intrinsically more necessary than other types of overhead. For example, when faced with the choice of installing an additional telephone for a clinician or an administrator, the choice is all too often in favor of the latter. This is perhaps understandable. Nonclinical personnel have a clear idea of their tasks, while they often have only a vague sense of the type of support clinicians require. Why, one might ask, do such situations arise? In the case of the telephone, as in many similar instances, it is little more than competition and the associated cognitive insularity that develops between groups within institutions.

## Information

Finally, government and corporate third-party payers have a clear interest in seeing to it that patients are fully informed about the details of their care. Patients who are not provided with this information in an understandable form are not in the position to cooperate to the degree that successful treatment requires. Poorly informed patients are more likely to become dissatisfied and to drop out of treatment at critical times. Unfortunately, for payers, the well-informed patient might begin to demand higher quality than the payers might wish.

## Insurance Companies

What, then, do insurance companies want? Or, to ask the question in a more relevant way, "What is it that insurance companies should not want?" Perhaps one of the least likely activities in which an insurance company ought to engage is day-to-day healthcare delivery. All the skills and instincts so necessary for successful pursuit of clinical care are absent; many of the dangers and pitfalls that defeat effective care delivery are present. At heart, insurance depends on reducing apparently dissimilar phenomena to accountable and interchangeable units. Medical care fundamentally depends on individual assessment and particularized intervention. Insurance companies must assume that the moral hazards for potential fraud are clear and present, while clinical care demands a measure of mutual trust and resists detailed accounting. The task of actuarial calculation is to reduce wildly dissimilar events to a final common path of money paid in compensation for unusual losses. The task of medical care is to come to grips with trouble, which, sooner or later, is certain to occur in all of us and to ameliorate the trouble with thoughtfulness, compassion, and the appreciation of individual differences. It is for these reasons that it is hard to imagine a human activity that is more lacking in congruence than insurance for run-of-the-mill medical care. Nevertheless, with the invention of managed care, this melding of purpose continues with the predictable result of increasing confusion and discord.

Insurance companies want a reasonable return of income on their investment of capital and labor. Publicly traded corporations depend on this rate of return on capital to encourage investors to buy their common stock. As there are many competing companies, each strives to have its "reasonable" return just a little bit higher than its competitors. To be the most successful, the corporation must exceed the average by a noticeable margin. The current expectation of insurance/managed care companies is that they should have about 60% "medical losses," or about 40% "reasonable" return. As competition puts pressure on these figures, more and more expenditures related to care must be moved from the "required" category and into the "elective" or optional realm.

Let us digress a moment and deal with what insurance company executives often say when asked about the 60%–40% figure. The 40% figure means that at least 40 cents of every insurance dollar goes to such things as administration, profits, and stock dividends. Insurance executives will sometimes argue that the 40% figure is justified because companies are reducing the administrative costs of providers and hospitals and because providers and hospitals are certain to be paid. Don't believe it. Hospital administrative costs have risen hand-in-hand with the administrative costs of insurance companies. In addition, on the subject of who is paid, only the insurance company is assured of being paid. Depending on circumstances and insurance company decisions, providers and hospitals may or may not be paid.

Insurance and managed care companies want satisfied subscribers. Yet it is important that some subscribers be more satisfied than others are. In fact, it is highly desirable that healthy subscribers be highly satisfied with their healthcare, while sick subscribers should be dissatisfied with the care, and the sicker, the more dissatisfied. Only then are the very sick likely to drop out and seek some type of healthcare coverage with a new carrier or the government. Far better, then, to increase the advertising budget in an effort to attract healthy new subscribers than to use these precious financial resources on the care of the sick who, it is hoped, will take their business elsewhere.

What this adds up to is the following. In a competitive environment, insurance companies must try to satisfy subscribers, but primarily the healthy ones. They must also satisfy stockholders, executives with expectations for high compensation, media critics, governmental regulators, and employees who expect high salaries and lavish benefits (such as healthcare), and somehow remain attractive to potential new members. That constant turmoil, decision changes, and deception have become the signature of many insurance companies providing health insurance is thus not surprising.[2]

Similarly, government at all levels brings a set of concerns and interests to bear when dealing with healthcare. As with insurance companies, some of these concerns are legitimate and proper, while others are less so. The first concern of any responsible government is to have a healthy population of workers, taxpayers, and voters. Governments are made of people, and these people, like everyone else, depend on a well-functioning system. All the activities of government work better when a population has the strength and productivity that good health brings. As health tends to promote productivity, so does productivity tend to promote a robust collection of taxes, the essential nutrient of governmental well-being. Finally, a healthy population in general) tends to imply that voters will be contented and thus be likely to smile on incumbency.

Nevertheless, the government, like corporations, has some interests of dubious social value. Most employees wish for advancement in their occupations, and for government, as for large corporations, this generally means increasing the size and complexity of the organization. The most certain route to higher status in a bureaucracy or a large corporation is to acquire the capacity to hire assistants. Because this is a tactic that is easily understood and emulated at every level, there exists a set of incentives to make all tasks appear as complicated and detailed as possible in order to justify the greater need for more personnel.

Just as the number of administrative positions has a relentless tendency to grow, so does the pressure for increased compensation. Corporations begin the process with the justification that the competitive environment requires that the most skilled personnel are hired, and so their salaries must reflect their value. At the apex of this process is the chief executive officer (CEO) whose compensation package is decided by a "compensation committee" of his board of directors. In most cases, this committee is composed of CEOs of other corporations. Needless to say, they tend to view the need for a high salary for their colleague with an understanding frame of mind. Thus, we now find that many CEOs of major healthcare enterprises enjoy annual compensation packages on the order of millions of dollars. Should this seem excessive, critics are reminded that healthcare is a highly competitive business and the very best management talent is crucial to the success of the enterprise. Similar points apply to government. Here the justification runs along the following lines: government must compete with private industry for talented people and so total compensation must be roughly equivalent, at least for those levels below the very top of the scale.

Let us return to perverse incentives that are specific to insurance companies. One that has received little attention so far, but which has profound implication for the long term, is the possibility of genetic screening for inherited illness. Diagnostic technology is currently improving by leaps and bounds, making it possible to predict with increasing accuracy whether an individual may be unusually susceptible, for example, to heart diseases, cancer, or strokes. Because these represent the majority of serious illnesses that Americans are likely to encounter, knowledge of the presence of genetic risk factors would be of considerable importance to the individuals involved, so that they might take prudent preventive measures where possible. Insurance companies armed with the same knowledge would have every incentive to use these data for profit maximization, either by excluding individuals from coverage or charging risk-based premium surcharges. Indeed, some would argue that the insurance companies would have a fiduciary responsibility to their stockholders to use every technological enhancement to refine their actuarial calculations.

Another perverse incentive, amounting to a moral hazard, is the possibility of a direct correlation between corporate profit and deceptive practice. This might come about several ways. Let us say that two treatment styles or protocols are used for a particular illness. At first, neither has been shown to have clear superiority. One is cheap, and the other is expensive. So far, there is no moral problem—we all agree that cheaper is better for equivalent effectiveness. Let us also say that a group of physicians then proposes a study to determine which of the two treatment methods is superior. What benefit accrues to the corporation from the study? The cheap method is already being used. Suppose that the study shows a clear superiority for the expensive method? Should the insurance company sponsor the study? Is it possible that the company will even try to impede it? Would they allow the physicians on their payroll to participate? Might they insist that their physicians not discuss the expensive option with patients? This is, of course, the infamous "gag rule," by which some corporate providers have attempted to control the flow of information between healthcare professionals and patients in the service of profit maximization. As we are writing this chapter, the matter is still in dispute, with court challenges to the propriety of such rules. Court decisions or not, the practice is improper, and vitiates the whole idea of healthcare.

Another recent example of the cost problem concerns the debate about the proper use of antiviral drugs for patients stricken with HIV. Should a single (expensive) drug be used, or would a combination of three (very expensive) drugs be used? Should the treatment begin early, before the onset of major symptoms, or is it better to wait until the disease progresses? These are questions that can be answered to a point of moral certainty by the appropriate use of carefully designed clinical trials. One answer is true, and another is false.

Yet another example of corporate moral hazard has to do with the use of specialists. It is now often asserted by managed care corporations that the use of generalists is appropriate for a variety of conditions formerly treated by specialists. There is in fact little evidence to support this assertion. Moreover, this assertion has led to family practitioners or general internists being asked to diagnose and treat psychiatric illness, neurological conditions, complicated blood diseases, and many obscure medical problems. Nurses are being used to replace physicians. Nonlicensed personnel are being used in place of nurses. Is this always good? Does it even really save money? It is hard to argue that less training is equivalent to more training, especially in an area of work the essence of which is the application of individualized judgment.[3]

### Regulatory Bodies

Similar perverse incentives influence the perspectives of civil servants and members of regulatory bodies. One such body is the Joint Commission on Accreditation of Healthcare Organizations (JCAHO) which we discussed earlier. Here it will be given a closer look. JCAHO was organized more than four decades ago by the efforts of the American Medical Association, the American College of Physicians, the American College of Surgeons, and the America Hospital Association. The original charter was for this independent group to survey the performance of hospitals according to professionally mandated standards of appropriate care. The surveys were to be voluntary, and the costs were borne by the hospitals requesting survey for the coveted accreditation. The visiting surveyors were typically retired senior clinicians whose experience and advice could reasonably be sought by any good hospital. Standards were developed to assess quality of performance in maintenance of the physical plant, infection control, adequacy of staffing, mortality and morbidity rates, and many other ways of making quantitative judgments about the care being given.

This worked quite well at first. The hospitals were the clients of JCAHO, and accreditation was highly valued but not strictly necessary for the hospital to stay in business. The professionals and the hospitals retained considerable control of the criteria by which their performance and quality might be judged. There was every incentive for JCAHO to develop and apply standards that were widely recognized and agreed upon, and when they did so, there were reasonable checks and balances. The hospitals would take care not to depart too much from the standards, lest they be embarrassed by an admonition from JCAHO, but likewise, JCAHO needed to take care that its standards were reasonable.

As time went on, JCAHO began to travel down the all-too-frequently seen road toward autonomous bureaucracy. Staff of the central administration multiplied many times. More and more surveyors were needed, which meant of course that they were not always as expert as the professionals that they were advising. Standards multiplied in complexity. The voluntary nature of the surveys began to erode. Accreditation became mandatory, because government and other third-party payers began to require JCAHO approval before they would agree to reimbursement.

With accreditation now required, for practical purposes the equilibrium of power and the system of checks and balances deteriorated. No longer was it so clear that the hospitals were the clients of JCAHO. Standards that presumed to measure quality seemed to bear less and less relationship to the practical clinical tasks at hand. Regulations began to change without any obvious reason. Surveyors became less collegial and began to resemble proconsuls in a wayward colony. Every new management fad appeared in the ever-expanding manuals that were supposed to guide practitioners in understanding compliance with the standards. Hospital administrators who had the temerity to protest were waved aside with the sardonic comment that after all, accreditation was still "voluntary."

Thus, there developed a situation in which greater and greater fractions of institutional resources were diverted to jumping through the hoops of JCAHO rather than using management skills to solve real problems. When faced with the choice of a real quality improvement versus illusory ones that were covered by the standards, the choice was clear. Holding essentially absolute power over the institution's very existence, JCAHO has developed insularity and matching arrogance that has few equals in contemporary America.

This is not to say that JCAHO is unresponsive to the concerns of hospitals. It has developed an elaborate system to allow for practice surveys. Surveyors may be hired as consultants to the hospital. For a substantial fee, they will instruct clinicians and administrators in the ever-changing arcana of the standards. JCAHO publishes instruction manuals that it earnestly urges the hospitals to buy. Then the actual survey comes, a traumatic event that throws the entire institution into frenzy. After three or four or five days (their choice) of hosting two to five surveyors, there is an exit conference that all interested parties are expected to attend. There the surveyors comment upon the quality that they have observed. Weeks later, the official pronouncement comes from the central offices of JCAHO that the hospital has passed with commendation, passed, conditionally passed with the requirement that certain perceived deficiencies will be corrected in a timely manner, or failed. To assure that corrections are made, another ad hoc survey may be ordered (of course at the expense of the hospital).

Let's get this straight now. JCAHO is an independent organization that has the power to force closure of healthcare organizations if it judges that certain of its standards are not met. The organizations it evaluates have negligible input into the development of the standards and they must bear the costs of the surveys, the intensity and frequency of which are determined by JCAHO, which sells its consulting services to this captive audience. There is no clear feedback mechanism to assure that the biases of JCAHO bear any genuine relationship to quality. The message is clear: go along with us and be accredited, or argue and fail. Pay whatever we ask, as often as we ask, and be grateful.

JCAHO is not the only regulatory authority, of course. There are federal and state governmental oversight agencies as well. Standards from each must be met by hospitals, for each has the power to cause them to have to cease operations. This is, in general, not unreasonable, but there are situations in which the standards required by one are not clearly compatible with another, with JCAHO, or often with quality healthcare.

## CONCLUDING COMMENTS

What can we conclude from this chapter concerning the development of a better healthcare system? We should keep firmly in mind that healthcare is fundamentally a transaction between patients and professional providers of knowledge and skill. Governments and insurance companies have a place, to be sure, but their functions are ancillary to the main task. Patients and providers should lead the process, and governments and insurance companies should facilitate the transactions and not presume to have the wisdom to direct them. As to oversight and audit committees, they too have their function, but if quality, highly accessible, low-cost healthcare is their objective, their function cries for drastic change.

## NOTES

1. J. Kleinke, writing in *Barron's*, 22 December 1997, considers what he calls "managed care meltdown"—a fundamental paradox at the heart of the HMO concept that the more an HMO invests in its members' health, the less its profit. That this obvious truth had remained obscure for so long illustrates the capacity of the public for denial, the failure to understand the nature of incentives, or the skill of HMO marketers in hiding the truth.

2. An additional difficulty is that until recently insurance companies and HMOs have been relatively insulated from liability for which they have been the proximate cause. However, L. McGinty has reported in the *Wall Street Journal*, 12 January 1998, that there is now increased interest in the concept that HMOs might properly be held liable for treatment coverage denials.

3. Moral hazards appear to be everywhere. N. Jeffrey, *Wall Street Journal*, 23 December 1997, reports that the American Association of Retired Persons (AARP), after criticism for a conflict of interest, has decided not to make endorsements of HMOs. There had been an initiative to require HMOs to pay a $20 fee *per month* to AARP for each member enrolled under the program.

*Part III*

# The Missing Parts of US Healthcare

*Chapter 8*

# Individual Human Nature— Healthcare's Missing Link

As hard as I try I can't escape the feeling that today's medicine is hostile.
. . . I have the best healthcare insurance around. . . . But it doesn't matter. . . . Getting an appointment is a major undertaking—it takes at least
a half-dozen calls . . . and a routine appointment can eat up half a day.
. . . Then there is the wait and uncertainty when procedures need to be
approved. . . . My husband has cataracts—they're so bad he no longer
drives. . . . Three doctors—they don't work for the insurance companies—agree that he needs surgery . . . but the insurance company says
"No!"—they refuse to approve the procedure. They say he's not ready
for the operation yet.

> Interview with a 45-year-old married mother of
> five children, university graduate with a Ph.D. in
> biology, and a tenured university faculty member

## INTRODUCTION

Thus far, we have discussed healthcare myths, the state of US healthcare,
and healthcare from the perspectives of patients, providers, and payers. What
has not been done is to look at the behaviors that patients, providers, and
payers have in common. To turn to these behaviors is to enter the domains
of individual and group human nature; that is, the behavior of individuals
and groups that tends to occur no matter what one's sex, social class, economic state, ethnicity, role, job, or political affiliation. These behaviors form
the bedrock on which any healthcare system, good, bad, or otherwise must
build. If existing healthcare systems are to be understood, and tomorrow's
healthcare systems are to be improved over today's, individual and group

human nature will need to assume their rightful positions at center stage of healthcare planning and implementation. This chapter is about individual human nature. Group human nature is the topic of Chapter 9.

## ECONOMIC, SOCIOLOGICAL, AND PSYCHOLOGICAL VIEWS

There is more than one lens through which to view individual behavior. Depending on the lens that is selected, both the behavior that is observed and its explanations differ. The economic lens focuses on individuals as players in the marketplace where material costs and benefits are the critical factors influencing behavior. The sociological lens substitutes culture, tradition, and social values for material costs and benefits. The psychological lens gives priority to the structure and content of information and the ways in which they shape behavior.

At first pass, these approaches might seem to provide the essential perspectives for understanding the workings of past and future healthcare systems. At second pass, one is less sure. Five decades of unsatisfactory solutions to healthcare suggests that the economic, sociological, and psychological views, alone or in combination, lack critical perspectives to guide healthcare planners through murky waters.

What is missing from these views? Before answering this question, it needs to be underscored that costs and benefits, culture, and information are very much a part of today's healthcare systems, just as they will be of future systems. Healthcare is about two persons making and effectuating decisions about the body, mind, and behavior of one of the participants. There are explicit and implicit contracts as well as expectations in such interactions. Some, but far from all, of the details of such interaction can be informed by economic analyses such as an HMO's response to costly patients. Sociological analyses can help explain many of the attitudes and preferences that patients and providers bring to healthcare encounters. The same point applies to psychology, where language and education influence what information is valued and how it is processed. Still, these factors address only part of the interaction story. Moreover, should we rely primarily on economic, sociological, and psychological insights to guide us through revisions of our healthcare system, the job will not get done. An appreciation of the fundamentals of human behavior and how these fundamentals relate to healthcare needs to move to center stage.

## EVOLUTIONARY BIOLOGY

Where does one look to find out about these fundamental behaviors? Who has done research? Who has talked about them? Who has written about them? The answers to these questions is evolutionary biologists.

Readers may imagine that evolutionary biology is an esoteric academic pastime, concerned primarily with the features and the strategies of survival and reproduction among nonhuman species and the changes in these strategies over time. Until the late 1920s, this view was more or less accurate. Things took a turn in the 1930s, however, when evolutionary biologists turned their attention to the evolution of *Homo sapiens.* The intervening decades have witnessed a myriad of insights about why human beings behave as they do and the factors that influence their behavior. Not only do these insights help explain many of the successes and failures of past and present healthcare systems, but they also can serve as a map for developing healthcare solutions in the future. For example, it is not necessary to teach emotions to children, to teach them to avoid pain or to like sweets, to teach them anger at being cheated, to teach them motivation to get what they want, or to teach them to take a keen interest in the opposite sex during adolescence. These behaviors come naturally. Further, individuals learn certain things easily, such as one's first language, while learning many other things, such as playing the piano well, is difficult. They respond emotionally to certain types of personal loss. And they will often deceive and self-deceive, yet they are only moderately successful at detecting others' deceptions.

These behaviors occur because human beings are predisposed to think, feel, and behave in specific ways. These ways have evolved through time. The source of these predispositions is our genes, just as the sources of our ears, our noses, and our circulatory systems are in our genes. Predispositions both influence and constrain behavior in predictable ways, and because literally all individuals share essentially the same predispositions, they have the effect of leveling the behavior playing field.

Interesting as it might be, it would be prohibitive to discuss all of the known or likely predispositions that guide and constrain human behavior. What can be achieved is to look at those key predispositions that have in the past and will in the future come into play with any healthcare system. These include personal survival, trust, reproduction, kin investment, reciprocal altruism, self-interest, cooperation, free riders, uncertainty reduction, and trait variation. Together, they explain the fundamentals of human behavior—behavior that is only partially refined and influenced by economic, sociological, and psychological factors.

## PERSONAL SURVIVAL

There is nothing unfamiliar about the idea that human beings act in ways to increase their chances of survival. From the early moments of life until death, people attempt to avoid dangerous and painful situations, to eat when they are hungry, to rest when they are tired, and to seek help when they are ill. That the number of years the average person is expected to live continues to rise as our capacities to combat diseases improves is what would be expected if there is a predisposition to survive. There are exceptions of course. Some adolescents drive dangerously and die because they do. Some individuals commit suicide. Some adults consume excessive amounts of alcohol and kill their livers. Still, the vast majority of individuals do not engage in these behaviors excessively. Moreover, with the exception of the occasional person who is intent on suicide, those who drive dangerously, drink or smoke excessively, or fail to exercise and eat correctly are thankful if their lives can be prolonged.[1]

The healthcare implications of survival are straightforward. Patients will seek out providers because they want to survive; they will reject those providers that they believe are not interested in their survival. The same points apply to providers and third parties. They will also act to survive.

## TRUST

Healthcare providers are ethically committed to prolonging survival. Patients will expect them to act to do so. More is involved here than the doctor and the patient agreeing that they share the same goal, however. For a large number of patients, their willingness to engage in behavior that increases their survival possibilities (e.g., stop smoking, increase exercise, reduce the intake of fats) is determined by their trust in providers. Much of the treatment side of healthcare amounts to educating and persuading patients to engage in certain proactive behaviors and following medical recommendations. A provider may occasionally scare a patient into a new lifestyle, yet more effective and lasting behavioral changes occur when provider and patient trust one another and both understand that the patient's survival is the basis for their interaction.

Trust is not something that magically graces every relationship, medical or otherwise. Nor is it an inevitable outcome of growing up. Rather, there is a predisposition to trust that must be nurtured if it is to influence behavior significantly. At the very least, nurturance requires that parents engage in loving and supportive relationships with their children and that, when children grow up, they have friends and family who are trustworthy. Applied to healthcare, trust necessitates honest communication between provider and patient. It is necessary that they cooperate in the context of a shared goal. Honesty and cooperation must persist over time and through multiple encounters. These requirements suggest a set of common sense guidelines applicable to both patients and providers. If trust is to develop, continuity of care, open communication, and sensitivity to what each party brings to interactions are essential. If either party is incapable of controlling continuity—this is often a reality at clinics or inpatient facilities where providers rotate—trust is endangered. When providers are constrained from open communication, as often happens when they work for insurance companies or HMOs, trust can become a rare commodity.

## REPRODUCTION

There is also nothing surprising about the fact that males and females are predisposed to reproduce, that the majority of males and females want to have offspring, or that the majority do so. The desire to reproduce is as much a part of human nature as is the aversion to pain. Again, there are exceptions. Some individuals do not want children. Some are unable to reproduce. Some start to have offspring but change their minds. Exceptions do not prove rules, but rather, they make them.

Patients will expect healthcare providers to facilitate healthy and satisfying reproduction. Trust is a critical variable if this outcome is to be achieved. Women are sensitive to who examines them physically and to the thoughtfulness of the medical recommendations they receive. This point applies particularly to difficult pregnancies where close medical monitoring is critical to the life of the fetus and the mother. Provider sensitivity, continuity of care, and the ability of providers to make optimal reproduction-relevant decisions are all contributing factors to developing trust and improving the health of mother and child. Patients' honesty, their willingness to follow medical recommendations, and their contributions to clarity and efficiency in patient–provider interactions make up the other half of the health equation.

## KIN INVESTMENT

Kin investment is a term evolutionary biologists use to refer to the predisposition of individuals to invest their time and resources preferentially in persons to whom they are related genetically. We may feel that some of the children who live down the street are more attractive and more intelligent than our own offspring, but rarely do we invest more time and energy in these children than in our own. So also with our brothers, sisters, nieces, nephews, and cousins. On average, they will receive more of our attention and resources than will all but our closest nonkin friends.[2]

Relatives will expect providers to act to enhance the survival and reproductive chances of kin that are ill. Most providers know this and will attempt to meet the expectations. Such expectations carry very specific implications for providers, including thoroughness of care, precise communication to relatives about the possible consequences of diseases and interventions, as well as recommendations about the length of convalescence. Trust is not absent in kin investment. Both providers and patients are usually aware of the need for trust when relatives are involved, particularly so when a healthy relative is responsible for carrying out medical recommendations for an ill child or an aging parent.

## SELF-INTEREST, COOPERATION, RECIPROCAL ALTRUISM, AND FREE RIDERS

It is an axiom of evolutionary biology that human beings act in their own self-interest, not in the interest of the group. *But pause before jumping to conclusions about this axiom.* Self-interested behavior does not necessarily equate with selfish, narcissistic, deceptive, or noncooperative behavior. Rather, it means that an estimate of the personal consequences and benefits of an act will influence the probability of an act. More important, self-interested acts can often turn out to have win-win outcomes. A patient who communicates openly and follows medical recommendations is likely to benefit through improved health, which, in turn, may benefit a spouse, relatives, friends, and providers. A mother's thoughtful and loving care for her child may be self-interested behavior on the part of the mother, yet her child stands to benefit. A provider's care for a patient is also self-interested behavior. The patient benefits from quality care and the provider benefits from the patient's response, an enhanced reputation, and increased financial security.

Win-win is not the only outcome of medical encounters, however. If a patient is untruthful—this often happens when persons suffer from mental illness or abuse substances—the provider may entertain the wrong diagnosis or make the wrong medical recommendation and thus inadvertently participate in a lose-lose situation. Or in situations in which a provider is primarily concerned with financial rewards or adhering to the constraints imposed by his or her employing organization, then the probability of quality medical decisions and recommendations declines. *It follows that one of the keys to developing a successful healthcare system is to increase the probability that encounters will have win-win outcomes rather than win-lose or lose-lose outcomes.*

If everyone is self-interested, then it might seem that this behavior would apply equally to all persons at all times and thus to any type of healthcare system. If this were the case, there would be no need to include self-interest in the healthcare equation. Yet nothing could be further from the truth. There is far more to developing win-win outcomes than occasionally helping one's neighbor jump-start his car and being rewarded with a free ride to work. Experience tells us that the degree to which individuals cooperate is influenced by a variety of factors. As might be expected, there are many lenses through which to examine these factors. Sociologists view cultural values as well as the explicit and implicit rules of group behavior as important factors influencing the likelihood of cooperation. Psychiatrists and psychologists tell us that psychological maturity and recognition of the fact that *no man is an island unto himself* are prerequisites for increasing the chances of win-win outcomes. Religious leaders provide moral interpretations. The more one considers others and the more one acts in their interest, the more one acts in the image of God and the more likely will be cooperative outcomes. Economists and businessmen argue that win-win outcomes are primarily influenced by marketplace incentives; human beings are inclined to try to win at the expense of others, but they can also spot a good bargain, and if the bargain is right, cooperation may follow.

Each of these views has its adherents and some supporting evidence. For example, some societies have more cooperators than other societies. Cultures that systematically honor and reward cooperators as well as punish noncooperators have a higher frequency of cooperation than cultures such as the United States in which honor and reward are sporadic. These points notwithstanding, a closer analysis of the preceding explanations of cooperation reveals a host of contradictions. For example, economic imperatives, such as "Shop around and get the best deal you can for yourself," often conflict with social values, such as "Buy American," or religious values, such as "Do unto others as you would have others do unto you."[3]

If sociological, psychological, and economic explanations of cooperation leave much to be desired, where might we turn to get a better understanding of cooperation and the conditions that influence it? Again, insights provided by evolutionary biologists provide both novel and critical insights.[4]

It is easy enough to understand why kin will cooperate to improve each other's health. They share genes, resources, and (often) values. However, shared genes and common interests in resources do not explain cooperation among nonkin. Reciprocal altruism refers to the bi-directional helping among two persons that are not genetically related by common descent, that is, friends. Nearly everyone has friends that one helps and who help in return. Such relationships are important if only because they offer opportunities that kin often can not or do not provide, such as sharing interests or assisting one another in careers.

Reciprocal altruism refers to exchanges that are separated in time. For example, I watch over my neighbor's dog while the neighbor takes a trip and several weeks later my neighbor helps me paint my barn. The time interval between help and payback differentiates this form of behavior from mutualism, a behavior in which two or more individuals help one another simultaneously and in which the costs and benefits to each are both apparent and approximately equal. Reciprocal altruism is central to our discussion because the most fundamental encounters of day-to-day healthcare are non-kin interactions that take place between patients and healthcare personnel. Although there are exceptions, such as risking one's life to help unknown others who are endangered (a truly selfless behavior), reciprocal altruism occurs most frequently and predictably when the benefits from helping others are likely to equal or to exceed the costs of helping. The "equal or to exceed" part of the equation depends on a number of factors.[5]

One factor is the degree to which participants know each other, particularly their past histories as reciprocators. Individuals tend to help others who they know and who have a history of reciprocating. They are less likely to help persons who they do not know or who have a history of failing to reciprocate. Such behavior is understandable. Few of us like to give repeatedly without receiving something in return.

Another factor is the degree to which players understand the "currency" of helping and repayment. No two reciprocal exchanges are ever quite the same. For example, a person may watch over his neighbor's house and collect the mail while the neighbor is away, and the neighbor may repay the helping with a timely stock market tip or a dinner at a restaurant. Most of the time both parties understand that the helping has been repaid. How is this possible? The most parsimonious explanation is that humans have a predisposed capability for making complex cost–benefit calculations that translate different behaviors into a common currency. Clearly, understanding the currencies that are pertinent to healthcare interactions becomes a critical issue when examining the ways in which exchanges between providers and patients take place in healthcare systems.

At this point, a cynic might ask, "Why don't more individuals defect in reciprocal relationships?" The question is important. A fact of life is that some people do defect. They receive from others and then disappear. Yet most do not. Moreover, fewer defect if there are clear social consequences from failing to reciprocate. Effective and efficient social consequences work best when there is a tightly knit social community in which participants are known to each other and where information about nonreciprocation travels rapidly throughout the community.

Avoiding the social consequences of failing to reciprocate is one of the critical motivating factors of human behavior. The doctor who fails to reciprocate (e.g., communicate precisely) with his or her patients invites rejection, complaints, and noncompliance with his or her medical recommendations. Likewise, the patient who fails to reciprocate (e.g., follow medical recommendations) invites medical inattention. When person–person encounters are impersonal, that is when it is unlikely that a patient will again encounter the provider with whom she or he is interacting, there are usually few social consequences for nonreciprocation. This is often the case in healthcare systems where providers rotate. In effect, social constraints that function to encourage persons not to defect from a reciprocal exchange are absent and thus difficult to enforce. On the other hand, when social constraints are present and they are enforceable, those who defect have a reduced chance of receiving quality healthcare in the future.

Discussions of reciprocal altruism go hand-in-hand with the topic of free riders. With good reason, evolutionary biologists have long argued that any society will contain a percentage of persons who do not reciprocate and engage in deceptive or default behavior. "Free riders" is the name often given to such persons. They make promises they do not keep. They deceive. And they accept help from others but fail to return it.

Unfortunately, and no matter what the precautions or social enforcements, any system will have its share of free riders. Healthcare systems are not exceptions. Some patients provide inaccurate information to obtain drugs. Some refuse to pay their medical bills. Some providers and hospitals charge for services they have never rendered. Some HMOs and insurance companies systematically bilk Medicare and Medicaid. Free riding will not go away. The questions are, Can it be contained? and What are the costs of containment?

Scientists estimate that under the best of conditions at least 5% of the individuals in any society are free riders. The 5% figure applies to social groups in which reciprocal altruism is an important social value and social ostracism is an effective way of constraining deception and defection. *In literally all instances*, this means small groups where group members know each other personally, particularly each other's reciprocation histories. When groups increase in size, when individuals do not know each other well, and when word-of-mouth communication does not extend to all members of the group—large city hospitals are an example—then social ostracism has far less impact on the behavior of free riders. In these circumstances, the percentage of free riders will increase. Patients, providers, administrators, and payers will all have their share.

Free riders are costly to healthcare systems and the costs are usually discussed in terms of dollars, as are instances in which medical bills are unpaid or oversight groups measure medical fraud. Yet the more destructive effects on healthcare are not quickly translated into dollars. Because free riders consume time and resources, they often deprive others of timely care, and in turn, they reduce morale and trust among healthcare providers and payers.

Reducing the number of free riders, which means attempting to approach the 5% level without incurring prohibitive costs, thus becomes an issue with significant economic and quality-of-care implications. Said another way, it is the motivation to develop and maintain healthcare systems in which there are social consequences for failing to reciprocate that will largely determine the degree to which healthcare systems can be optimized. Said yet another way, cooperation can be the modus operandi of patients and healthcare systems alike. If patients, doctors, nurses, and healthcare administrators cooperate, then high-quality, cost-efficient, user-satisfying healthcare systems are a possibility. If they fail to do so, we will have more of what we have now—that is, fits and starts with far from satisfactory solutions.

## INTERACTION UNCERTAINTY

All species act to reduce uncertainty, *Homo sapiens* included. Uncertainty reduction is one of the reasons we interact with the same persons time and time again rather than rarely interacting with the same person twice. Why is reducing uncertainty so important? There are a number of easy answers to this question. One is that uncertainty is frightening. It causes anxiety, worry, and fear. Another is that it often reduces one's ability to concentrate. Still another is that one's decisions are often off the mark and cooperation with others is less likely.

In both known and unexpected ways, uncertainty creeps into literally every facet of healthcare. Diagnoses and test results may be ambiguous and uninformative. Patients may give conflicting histories. Guidelines for clinical conduct may be imprecise or not relevant to many commonly encountered medical situations. Medical bills may be difficult to interpret. In addition, drugs may have unexpected and adverse side effects. Yet, within limits, uncertainty can be reduced. Interpersonal uncertainty can be minimized by making plans, establishing and following guidelines, interacting with persons who have a proven record of acting on their word, and by establishing trust. These points apply equally to patients and healthcare providers.

Still, even with the best of efforts at uncertainty reduction, there will be hitches, and the most important hitch is that illness introduces uncertainty into the lives of those who are ill as well as those who care for the ill. Patients will attempt to decrease their concerns about disease, healthcare costs, and their earning potential when they interact with healthcare providers. Ideally, healthcare providers will reduce both their own and their patient's uncertainty through providing accurate diagnoses, intelligent intervention strategies, and guidance. If uncertainty is high and cooperation is low, these events are unlikely to happen.

## TRAIT VARIATION

To this point in the chapter, we have focused on behaviors that are common to literally all individuals. We now turn and look at another feature of behavior. Trait variation is about individual differences. Some persons are more responsive to pain that others. Some are more predisposed to illnesses. Some reciprocate more than others do. Some lack capacities to care for themselves while others are capable of doing so. Some patients are more likely than others to comply with medical recommendations. Essentially the same points may be made about providers. Some are better diagnosticians than others. Some are more empathetic than others. Some work harder. Some care about their patients more.

Like every feature of human nature mentioned above, individual differences are not going to go away. They can be influenced but not eliminated by education. They don't disappear if there are laws against them. Most important for this book, individual differences pose significant problems for the design of healthcare systems. Consider the two extremes. Systems that attempt to standardize—"digitalize" is perhaps a better term—their approach to healthcare will increase the possibility that providers will be insensitive to many of the individuals they treat, that many patients will be dissatisfied, and that the quality of care will be far less than is desirable or possible. On the other hand, systems that attempt to individualize their approach to healthcare will increase the quality of care and reduce insensitivity to patients, but costs will increase. We offer a solution to this dilemma in Chapter 11, but the fundamental points may be set forth here. (a) Those healthcare systems that will survive will be responsive to individual differences. (b) Those that fail to survive will be unresponsive to individual differences. (c) The factor that will most distinguish the survivors from the nonsurvivors will be the degree of cooperation among the essential players.

## CLOSING COMMENTS

We have devoted much of this chapter to the topics of cooperation and reciprocal behavior. To review, these behaviors influence literally every facet of healthcare. Survival and kin investment influence how one interfaces with providers. Cooperation occurs more often among those who know each other compared to those who do not. Patients will support healthcare systems that reciprocate—that is, systems that provide quality and timely services for one's healthcare investment. Continuity of care thus becomes a desirable requirement for healthcare systems that seek to develop a cooperative ambiance. The currencies of helping and repayment differ across every facet of healthcare. For example, providers attempt to develop accurate diagnoses and to design optimal interventions, and patients are expected to give accurate information, to follow medical recommendations, and to pay for the services they have received.

Some readers may feel that we have overemphasized the importance of cooperation. For example, it can be argued that if economic incentives are sufficient, providers may be willing to diagnose and develop optimal interventions irrespective of whether or not patients cooperate. Likewise, with insurance companies and HMOs may be willing to remain in the healthcare business as long as they are making their desired profit. Yet to argue this way is to blind oneself to two critical points—one dealing with the quality of healthcare, the other with what is human. Concerning quality, healthcare involves far more than economic incentives. Critical components are morale, emotional support, reduction of fear and uncertainty, familiarity between patients and providers, trust, intervention timeliness, and an understanding that individual differences are as much a part of healthcare as dollars. Turning to what is human, cooperation tends to breed cooperation and high degrees of cooperation result in different outcomes and products compared to outcomes that result from economic incentives alone or from systems in which the percentage of free riders is high. It is these points that are absent in discussions about governmental or marketplace solutions to our healthcare problems. At times, these discussions assume that cooperation is not an issue. At other times they assume that cooperation follows from providing a service. That such thinking is folly is the logical conclusion from the history of welfare, the blight of much urban housing development, insurance company fraud, and HMO and insurance company rejections of legitimate medical claims. Without cooperation by all the players—and we are all players—optimal healthcare systems will remain an illusion.

## NOTES

1. See, for example, C. Ansberry, *Wall Street Journal*, 31 December 1997, in which he discusses findings from a survey indicating that most seniors accept limits of time and derive satisfaction with their elderly state. Some think it is the best period of their lives.

2. For a classic paper on kin investment see W. D. Hamilton, "The Genetic Evolution of Human Behavior," *Journal of Theoretical Biology* 7 (1964): 173–191.

3. For a classic research study dealing with the conditions that influence helping behavior, see S. Essock Vitale and M. T. McGuire, "Women's Lives from an Evolutionary Perspective: 2. Patterns of Helping," *Ethology and Sociobiology* 6 (1985): 155–173.

4. For an article examining the evolutionary conditions that might have favored the development of predispositions for magnanimity, see J. L. Boone, "The Evolution of Magnanimity," *Human Nature* 9 (1998): 1–21.

5. For a classic paper dealing with reciprocal altruism, see R. D. Trivers, "The Evolution of Reciprocal Altruism," *Quarterly Review of Biology* 46 (1971): 35–57.

*Chapter 9*

# Group Human Nature

If I didn't have a wife and three children I'd quit. . . . Maybe 30% of my time is spent treating patients . . . the rest is dealing with paperwork, ridiculous administrative meetings run by persons who can only think in terms of dollar signs, and fighting with uneducated jerks that determine the amount of care to be provided. . . . There is no way that I would submit my family to the kind of care we offer here.

Interview with a 38-year-old physician working for an HMO

## INTRODUCTION

If human beings are predisposed to act to survive, reproduce, invest preferentially in kin, and develop reciprocal relationships with selected nonkin, what about our behavior in groups in which the vast majority of the members are nonkin? This chapter is about behavioral predispositions and groups, the functions of groups, the reasons why individuals join groups, and the influence of group size on behavior and quality of care. We begin with some historical points.

## WORLD WAR II TO THE PRESENT

Prior to World War II, the trademark of American medicine was the individual doctor managing a private office. True, there were urban hospitals, community clinics, teaching hospitals, and Veterans Administration hospitals where large numbers of providers and supporting staff worked under a single roof. Nevertheless, the office of the individual doctor, perhaps supported by a nurse, was where the majority of medical encounters took place.

In the decades since World War II, the individual medical practitioner has largely disappeared so that today only a small percentage of providers work alone. Those that do are usually located in remote geographical areas or engage in highly specialized practices. A far larger percentage of providers work in groups varying in size from a few doctors, nurses, and technical/ support personnel to large groups composed of hundreds to thousands of members which, in addition to doctors, nurses, and technical/support personnel, include business managers, accountants, executives, and lawyers.

There are numerous reasons for these changes. As medical knowledge has increased, more minds have become necessary to master the details of medicine and to remain current with the latest diagnoses and treatments. New technical devices such as PET (positron emission tomography) and MRI (magnetic resonance imaging), analytic and diagnostic procedures (tissue analysis, DNA typing), and complex surgical techniques also have had their influence. The administration of PET and MRI to patients requires at least three trained individuals to conduct even the simplest of examinations as well as frequent visits by special technicians to keep the equipment in working order. Heart bypass surgery may require a team of a dozen individuals, each with his or her special expertise. Technical laboratories often require the expertise of a half-dozen individuals.

Few would fault the many technical, diagnostic, and treatment advances that have occurred since World War II. Organ transplants, the early detection of cancer, laser treatments, and renal dialysis are only a few example of what, by literally any measure, are indices of medical progress that has patient-related benefits. Yet there are also downsides to this trend. As healthcare groups have increased in size, both the efficiency and quality of medical care have come into question. Much of medicine has become big business, which means that values important to business, not necessarily those of quality healthcare, have come to dominate healthcare distribution.

Patients are not happy either. For example, in California, 50% of the patients who obtain their medical coverage through HMOs or insurance companies are dissatisfied. They are irritated with the time and effort required for making appointments. They are unhappy about the ways providers communicate; and they are angry because of disallowed treatments. If they were medically knowledgeable, they would be dissatisfied with much of the treatment they receive. It is one of the ironies of our times that many individuals who pay for healthcare in advance through either insurance premiums or HMO membership have to beg to obtain treatment and demand to be treated with respect.

At this moment in time, there is no indication that the trend towards bigness will change. Literally all the current blueprints for tomorrow's medicine assume that provider groups will be composed of large numbers of members and operate primarily as businesses or extensions of government— witness, for example, the "Clinton health plan." Moreover, despite the hype and promises, as we have argued, the introduction of the business mentality into medicine is not promising. Put in the form of a question, "Is bigness or the business mentality likely to solve America's healthcare needs in ways that improve quality of care, contain costs, and increase patient satisfaction?" One would have to be an incurable optimist to answer this question yes.

Now, to a closer look at groups.

## PREDISPOSITIONS AND GROUPS

Do behavioral predispositions still influence our actions when we are group members? Or are other factors more important? The answers to these questions are not difficult. Predispositions influence behavior in groups in the same way they do in one-to-one relationships. However, the importance of predispositions differs because groups often have different functions than do two-person interactions. These differences influence how one behaves. Consider the case of the working mother with three young children. At home, she will invest much of her time and energy in her offspring. She will feed them, take them to school, keep them clean, arrange birthday parties, and so forth. The same mother managing a small business will spend her time and energy in different activities, such as designing future company products, talking to potential customers, reviewing financial statements, deciding whom to hire or fire, and giving specific instructions to the sales staff.

Nowhere are the preceding points more applicable than in healthcare. The country doctor and his patients, HMOs with their cadre of providers and administrators, insurance companies with their large administrative staffs and gatekeepers, disease interest groups and their public relations staffs, and large university hospitals with their faculties and students will each have its unique group behavioral profile and set of priorities. Healthcare is in part about these profiles and their functions and in part about interactions between different profiles, efficiency, cost, and quality of care.

## GROUP FUNCTIONS

Because groups vary in their behavioral profiles and their functions, the degree to which members devote energy to group goals as well as the requirements for continuing group membership differ. Table 9.1, which compares features of hunter-gather groups with groups typical of Western urban society, illustrates these points.

There are clear functional differences distinguishing the two types of groups in Table 9.1. Compared to Western urban groups, members of hunter-gatherer groups share a greater commonality of purpose, engage in more kin-and group-related behavior, and have different group-related responsibilities. The most informative differences, however, are found in the attitudes of hunter-gatherers toward work, in their egalitarian and integrated

Table 9.1
Behavioral Differences among Hunter-Gatherer and Western Urban Groups

| | Hunter-Gatherer Groups | Western Urban Groups |
|---|---|---|
| Composition of the home | Extended family | Alone or nuclear family |
| Responsibility of individuals | Mainly to group | Mostly to individual |
| Work | Often enjoyable | Frequently disliked |
| Shared benefits | Agreed and integrated | Often disputed |
| Ceremonies | Regular and collective | Few, often meaningless |

*Source*: Adapted from *ASCAP (Across-Species Comparisons and Psychopathology)*, 10 February 1997. Includes both historical information and findings from current anthropological studies.

distribution of benefits, and in the value they accord to ceremonies. These differences are signs of group solidarity, where individual members devote much of their time and effort to activities that both directly and indirectly enhance the well being of other group members. Positive attitudes towards work mean that group members believe their efforts will be valuable to more persons than themselves. The egalitarian and integrated distribution of benefits (often despite a scarcity of resources) means that, in certain circumstances, sharing has a higher priority than competitive success and individual advantage. And the respect of ceremonies reinforces the group's place and purpose in the world.

Table 9.1 should not be taken to suggest that hunter-gatherer groups are ideal or that they provide a ready-made model which Western urban groups or US healthcare systems should adopt. The table is introduced to illustrate that there are other ways to organize groups, that the way in which they are organized has behavioral implications, and that alternative ways of organizing groups are worth considering if one's intent is to design high-quality healthcare systems. What the hunter-gatherers teach us is that groups can function to the advantage of the vast majority of their members, and not just a selected few. They can minimize certain forms of competition if these interfere with a common purpose. They can focus on the egalitarian distribution of benefits in preference to differential distribution. An obvious implication of these points is that our healthcare system has the option to live by different values and priorities. Moreover, arguably healthcare is the most obvious and important place where a new set of values and commonalties of purpose could have significant health, social, and financial consequences.

## WHY INDIVIDUALS JOIN GROUPS

Individuals join groups for different reasons. Group membership may increase an individual's financial and employment opportunities. It may offer preferential access to information. It may permit an individual to use special skills. The list of reasons is almost endless. Because it is, a reasonable premise is that no two persons join groups for exactly the same reasons. There is one important exception, however, and it concerns predispositions to achieve physiological and psychological well being—"homeostasis" is the medical term for this state of being. People who join groups do so in part to assure that they sustain homeostasis.[1]

Persons in this state feel healthy. They are motivated. They are able to think clearly and act efficiently. They participate. And they can tolerate periods of stress without adverse consequences. Those who are not in homeostasis feel less healthy. They are less motivated and less able to think clearly. They are less able to tolerate periods of stress. In addition, the chances that they will become bored, depressed, lonely, fearful, apathetic, and angry increase significantly.

How is homeostasis achieved? The answer is surprisingly straightforward. It is through engaging in specific types of social interactions and avoiding other types. Human beings are predisposed to interact in ways that balance our physiological and psychological systems. Social interaction, which means the exchange of thoughts and feelings, touching, helping, empathizing, and sex are as essential for this balance as air and glucose are for life.

For convenience, social interactions can be divided into those that are positive, those that are negative, and those that are neutral. Positive interactions occur when parents comfort a distressed child, when a wife comforts a husband fatigued from a hard day's work, when a friend provides guidance and support during difficulty times, and when a boss takes time to compliment an employee for a fine job performance. Positive interactions increase the chances of physiological and psychological balance. Negative social interactions involve the opposite kinds of behaviors, such as receiving unwarranted criticism, a friend rejecting a request for help, social ostracism, and a boss ignoring hard-working employees. Neutral interactions provide no indication whether another person has positive or negative feelings. Negative and to lesser degree neutral social interactions increase the chances of non-homeostatic states.

The physiological and psychological consequences of negative information are perhaps most obvious when one looks at how mothers interact with their offspring. A mother's holding, talking, and stroking will comfort a distraught nonhomeostatic child. Should a mother fail to provide this comfort, the child will become frustrated and eventually withdraw socially through exhaustion and sleep. In short, for infants and young children, specific types of interactions are essential if they are to remain physiologically and psychologically balanced. The same point holds for adults, although they sometimes claim otherwise. Adults need to be appreciated, respected, recognized, supported, and comforted. In the absence of such interactions, nonhomeostasis is likely.

The biological details of how interactions with others influence one's physiology and psychology are discussed in the medical literature and, with the exception of a few key points discussed below, this literature will not be surveyed here. What basically happens is this: positive and negative information from others influences chemicals in the brain (neurotransmitters) that are responsible for information transmission, thoughts, and feelings. Depending on the kind of information one receives, there will be either greater or fewer available chemicals to facilitate information processing and to initiate or dampen feelings. When the concentration of chemicals is optimal, one feels good and is in homeostasis. When the concentration is suboptimal (usually, below a certain level, but sometimes above), one feels bad and is imbalanced.

At first, the idea that information can influence brain chemicals may seem a bit farfetched. But consider a familiar example, such as the unexpected death of a loved one. One becomes depressed. Motivation declines. It is difficult to have fun or forget about the loss. Such changes are the direct consequences of chemical changes in the brain. Or take the instance where one has been rejected by a person one thought was a close friend. One may be depressed or angry. One may want to withdraw or retaliate. Alternatively, one may suddenly turn one's energies elsewhere in order to forget the rejection. Whatever the response, such events occur in part because of changes in the brain's chemical makeup.

What we are describing is analogous to the effects of different levels of glucose on feelings and thoughts. In the absence of the necessary amounts of glucose in one's blood and cells, one feels uneasy, has difficulty concentrating, and food becomes a preoccupation. When one obtains food, one feels better, concentration improves, and food is no longer a preoccupation. One has moved from a nonhomeostatic to a homeostatic state.

Figure 9.1 expands on the preceding points. Figure 9.1 shows the estimated increases in the amount of time spent grooming when our ancient ancestors are compared to modern humans. For nonhuman species, the term grooming usually refers to touching and cleaning other animals as well as certain ritual displays concerned with reproduction. Among human beings, it references a much wider array of behavior including talking with, recognizing, smiling at, touching, and helping others. At first glance, the figure of 40% grooming time for modern humans seems a surprisingly high percentage, particularly when one considers that the 40% means 24 of every 60

**Figure 9.1**
**Estimated Changes in the Time Spent Grooming across 3 Million Years of Evolution**

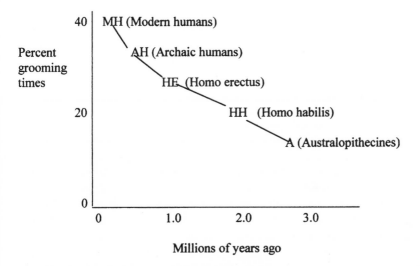

*Source*: R. Dunbar, *Grooming, Gossip, and the Evolution of Language* (Cambridge, MA: Harvard University Press, 1997).

waking minutes. Yet the 40% also invites an inquiry into why it is so high. Compared to our ancestors of hundreds of thousands of years ago, the evolution of modern humans appears to be characterized by increasingly strong predispositions to interact socially—for example, *Homo sapiens* show a 33% increase in grooming time over *Homo erectus*. Such increases do not appear without cause—that is, they are not random events. Rather, they reflect evolutionary outcomes that were adaptive for our ancestors. For today's humans, the main value of the predisposition to socialize is that it enhances the chances that we will remain social participants, not loners always fending for ourselves.

Because not all social interactions are positive, we adopt strategies when we interact with others. Countering our predisposition to interact is our predispostion to avoid interactions in which we feel we are unimportant and unneeded—that is situations in which others question our worth as group members. Moreover, we go to considerable lengths to avoid others that fail to recognize us or react to us negatively. Conversely, we go to considerable lengths to associate with persons who interact with us in positive ways and with whom we feel important, needed, worthwhile, and safe. We may explain our behavior in all kinds of ways, but maintaining a homeostatic state is the bottom line of such behavior. Like our desire to survive, reproduce, invest in kin, and maintain valued reciprocal relationships, our need to try to achieve homeostatic states is coded in our genes.

Homeostasis is of more than passing interest to healthcare. If a provider is bored, fearful, or socially withdrawn, the quality and efficiency of his or her work will decline. If patients are in nonhomeostatic states, which often happens when they are suffering from a disease, a disorder, or prolonged stress, they are less likely to participate in providing accurate histories or in carrying out providers' recommendations. And if healthcare administrators are nonhomeostatic, they will be less willing to devote their attention to developing quality and efficient healthcare systems.

Should one be skeptical about the preceding points, consider the following case history. A very distraught patient enters the emergency room of a hospital with an infection. The medical history reveals that the infection has been present for several weeks and that the patient has delayed seeking medical attention although he knew he should have done so. Given this history, the provider has a number of options. One is to chastise the patient for not seeking medical attention earlier and to proceed with treatment. Another is to disregard the fact that the patient delayed seeking help and proceed with treatment. Yet another is to accept the fact that the patient made a mistake and positively encourage him not to do so again. In the actual incident, the provider severely chastised the patient. Angered by the provider's response, and more distraught than when he arrived for treatment, the patient left the hospital before his infection was treated adequately. Two weeks later the patient died following the spread of the infection throughout his body.

## PATIENTS AS GROUP MEMBERS

Should patients be members of healthcare groups just as much as doctors, nurses, clinic managers, and administrators? We think so. Still, providers, third-party payer groups, even patients themselves rarely view things this way. Rather, patients tend to view themselves, and frequently are viewed by others, as individuals who receive services and provide revenue to providers. This is the service model of US business. It works well enough for such things as catering, plumbing, fast food outlets, and mail-order catalogue companies. Its relevance to healthcare is another matter.

Solutions to healthcare problems in part remain unsolved because patients think of themselves as nongroup members and others think of them as primary sources of revenue. When such thinking prevails, providers and third-party payers find it easier to rationalize increases in healthcare fees, to cut costs through limiting services, and to increase the distance between themselves and patients. They do this by making it difficult for patients to contact providers (gatekeeping), by disregarding patients' complaints, and by failing to provide appropriate information about healthcare coverage. In turn, it is the feeling of nonmembership that has been an important motivating factor among groups of patients and their relatives who join together in patient- and disease-advocacy groups and demand greater provider sensitivity to particular healthcare problems. Alzheimer's disease or diabetes groups are examples.

To argue this way is not to suggest that including patients as group members will solve all of our healthcare problems. Far from it. The fact that groups exist does not assure that groups will function in ways that predictably increase homeostatic states among their members or that groups will carry out their functions optimally. Group members often compete for power, discriminate against one another, play favorites, and socially ostracize innocent others. Yet, clearly, if patients were included as group members they would be less distraught and more homeostatic. Moreover, they probably would require less medical care and quality-of-care measures might improve.

## GROUP STRUCTURE

The preceding points invite a closer look at those features of groups that promote homeostatic and nonhomeostatic states. Four features can be singled out: group membership and common purposes; group membership and rule-following behavior; group membership and non–rule-following behavior; and group size.

The first two features (common or overlapping purposes and rule-following behavior) are relatively straightforward and require little additional explanation. Commonality of purpose, or shared objectives, directs members' energies in ways that can be advantageous to both patients and providers. Understanding the purpose of both explicit and implicit group-related rules—all groups have rules—and engaging in rule-following behavior is tantamount to saying that group members are aware of the advantages that can be gained for themselves as well as others when they adhere to a set of shared and understood behavioral expectations.

The third feature, that there are social consequences for non–rule-following behavior, was first addressed in Chapter 8. In that discussion, we emphasized that the *possibility* of social ostracism is a strong motivator to repay others' help and not to defect or cheat. Translated to healthcare, if reduced quality of care is likely to meet with disapproval by one's professional associates or the patients one treats, it is less likely to occur.

Advocating that social ostracism should be an integral part of the healthcare equation will raise the hackles of many. From one perspective, social ostracism seems cruel in that those who are ostracized pay both a psychological and physiological price, which means that their chance of becoming nonhomeostatic increases. Moreover, there are laws forbidding many types of ostracism. Employment practices require formal (e.g., written) warnings about one's behavior and specify appeals procedures if warnings or personnel decisions seem unjustified. From one perspective, it is difficult to argue with such laws because they often provide legal protections to individuals who have been unfairly treated. Are we not all familiar with situations in which the wrong people gain control of a group and ostracize those who are more responsible and talented? Such events occur.[2]

Yet to focus solely on possible inequities is to miss a more important and more salient point, namely the positive social and health effects can result when individuals act to avoid social ostracism for failing to meet adequate standards of quality delivery. Acting to avoid ostracism simply means acting in ways that meet the reasonable expectations that develop among group members. Such actions influence group behavior at a more fundamental level than biased or unfair employment procedures. Meeting reasonable expectations notifies others that one is a cooperator, that one can be trusted, and that one will act in ways that benefit persons other than the actor. Such notifications can be contagious, and when they are, homeostasis is the probable outcome. Two fundamental facts of life are that people make judgments and act on their judgments.

Equally important, when people work together, they engage in implicit contracts and expectations. Although a formal contract is never signed, the doctor who takes the time to enter a detailed history into a medical record reasonably expects that those who manage medical records will not lose them. The pharmacist who fills a prescription reasonably expects that the physician has written the correct prescription and that patients will take the medicine as directed. Again, no formal contracts are signed. Such transactions are based on implicit contracts. When expectations are not met, irritation, frustration, and anger often follow. Indeed, compared to the situation in which formal contracts are broken, irritation and frustration frequently are greater when implicit contracts are broken; and irritation at those who break contracts does not go away quickly.

Consider the following example. The quality of a provider's care begins to deteriorate in ways that are obvious to other group members. Other group members can either take notice or not. If they take notice and address the issue, they have increased the chances that the provider's care will improve. If they choose not to address the issue, then social ostracism is likely. In the former choice, the possibility of social ostracism is what initiates the change and nonhomeostatic states are avoided. In the latter, once ostracism has occurred, the chances of long, tedious, and often unproductive interactions increase significantly. To return to the facts of life, we treat people who irritate and endanger us differently than we treat people who support and protect us. Thus, from our perspective, the question is, "Can social ostracism be used effectively but not abusively to improve healthcare?" Our answer is yes, but only under certain conditions, one of the most important of which is group size.[3]

**Figure 9.2**
**Estimated Changes in Group Size across 3 Million Years of Evolution**

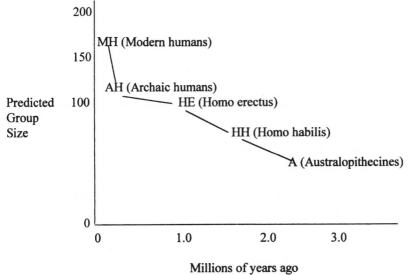

Source: R. Dunbar, *Grooming, Gossip, and the Evolution of Language* (Cambridge, MA: Harvard University Press, 1997).

## GROUP SIZE

The fourth feature that contributes to social environments that promote homeostasis is group size. The influence of group size is important enough to merit an in-depth discussion. For this reason, it is addressed here and from other perspectives in the next chapter. Group size has direct implications for quality of care and efficiency. HMOs, federal and state government agencies, medical associations, insurance companies, and large hospitals with multiple healthcare contracts are examples of groups that often have thousands of members. Evolutionary findings can provide insights into the relationships between group size, behavior, and quality of care. Figure 9.2 provides background information for this point.

Figure 9.2 plots the predicted average group size for modern humans and our ancestors dating back 3 million years. What the figure shows is that the upper limit of "naturally occurring" groups is approximately 160 persons, not several hundred or several thousand. Naturally occurring groups can be contrasted to what may be thought of as "artificial groups." The latter type of group is composed of many hundreds of individuals. These require the introduction of multiple structural features such as hierarchies to assure order, purpose, direction, and to facilitate communication.

No doubt our ancestors could have had larger groups. Perhaps they did and decided that they were undesirable. Whatever the details, they appear to have preferred to live in groups that did not exceed an upper limit. Why? There are several probable answers. One answer deals with how well members know each other—which, among other things, means how well reciprocation histories are known. The larger the group, the less detailed are the available histories. As the number of group members mounts, it becomes increasingly costly in terms of each member's time and energy to interact with unfamiliar individuals; on average, routine interactions with unfamiliar individuals require more time and energy than interactions with known individuals. A related consequence is that interaction uncertainty increases. Yet another consequence is that subgroups develop. This usually means that members of these groups will devote considerable time and energy to such things as establishing boundaries and acquiring privileges.

A second answer is that the larger the group the more difficult it is to identify free riders. As a result, increasing amounts of time and effort are spent trying to determine if others can be trusted, to divine their motives, and to decipher their communications. This is time and energy that could be devoted to more productive activities such as improving the efficiency with which the group operates and the quality of its products.

A third answer has to do with psychological and physiological homeostasis. As the number of group members increases, the probability of engaging in homeostatic interactions declines while the probability of neutral or negative communications increases. In large groups, members of one's preferred social network are often dispersed. When they are, grooming occurs less frequently than desired. In turn, individuals spend extra time seeking out those with whom they prefer to interact.

A fourth answer is that the positive effects of social ostracism decline.

As with Table 9.1, which contrasted functional behaviors of hunterer-gathers and Western urban society, Figure 9.2 is not introduced to suggest a model of group size that healthcare systems might blindly adopt. Nevertheless, there are lessons to be learned from Figure 9.2 in addition to those already discussed. Two are particularly important. The first deals with communication efficiency. Both the meaning and accuracy of what is communicated improves when groups are smaller. As groups increase in size, communication becomes more complex, more tedious, and the chances for misinterpretation increase—witness the inaccuracy of most gossip in large organizations. Largeness introduces a world in which face-to-face communication is replaced by job descriptions, manuals, letters, large group meetings, e-mail, rumors, faxes, and lawyers. The second deals with non–rule-following behavior. As groups become larger, there are consequences for rule-following behavior. Figure 9.3 illustrates what can happen.

In Figure 9.3, the frequency with which members guide their actions by a common set of rules declines as the number of persons in a group in-

**Figure 9.3**
**Estimated Effects of Group Size on Rule-Following Behavior among Group Members**

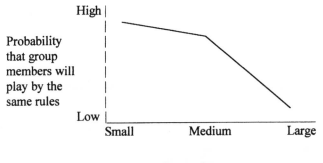

Group size

*Source*: Authors.

creases. The major decline in rule-following behavior occurs when groups exceed the medium size. Many of the reasons for the decline have already been noted. For example, the smaller the percentage of group members that are known to any individual, the more diverse the purposes of group members, and the greater the potential for conflict among members, then the more likely that subgroups with perverse incentives will form and act competitively with other subgroups. There is also the issue of interindividual accountability or the motivation of group members to self-monitor their own behavior. Self-monitoring is less effective as a group becomes larger. With a decline in the need to avoid social ostracism and in motivations to self-monitor, the number of free riders is likely to increase.

As groups increase in size, they try to develop ways of dealing with the increased difficulty of informally monitoring the behavior of their members. Formal accountability procedures, such as audits and complaint systems are initiated. Such systems are costly, time consuming, and of questionable effectiveness. They sap energy and resources that could be devoted to improving group efficiency and product quality. Hierarchical structures and review committees are put in place. Hierarchies have advantages, such as the assignment of persons with special skills to particular jobs where they can be most effective. Yet they also have disadvantages, such as the progressive distancing of management from many members of the group as well as from those persons whom the group is supposed to serve.

Patients and quality of care return to our discussion in Figure 9.4.

In the Figures 9.1, 9.2 and 9.3, patients were peripheral to the discussion. In Figure 9.4, they reenter the discussion. Figure 9.4 looks at what happens to quality of care among groups of different sizes. The figure shows that

**Figure 9.4**
**Estimated Changes in the Quality of Healthcare as a Function of Group Size**

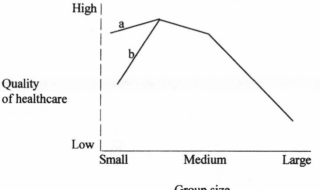

Group size

*Source*: Authors.

quality can vary among small groups. For those small groups that have a very limited healthcare focus, such as dentists, dermatologists, or ophthalmologists, small group size and quality-efficient care may go hand-in-hand. This outcome is represented by line *a* in Figure 9.4. However, a small group that attempts to deal with a wide array of medical problems presents another picture. The members of such groups are unlikely to have the necessary information and expertise to treat optimally a significant percentage of the medical conditions that they encounter. This outcome is represented by line *b* in Figure 9.4.

Figure 9.4 also suggests that the quality of healthcare will increase as the group size increases from small to medium. Compared to small groups, greater amounts of medical information and expertise are available in medium size groups, the upper limit of which we suggest is approximately 160 individuals. There are more crosschecks on diagnoses and treatment decisions. Medical mistakes are less likely. Quality improvement by informal internal monitoring is possible. And contingencies, such as sudden needs to provide emergency services, are manageable.

When groups expand beyond a certain size, the tendency is for quality of care to decline. From the patient's perspective, the increased probability of dealing with unfamiliar providers leads to uncertainty and anxiety. From the providers perspective, employees spend more time making certain that they will continue to survive in the organization for which they work (e.g., establishing and defending territories, attending mind-numbing administrative meetings, adjusting to new rules without knowing why they have been developed, pleasing those higher up in the organization). Employees also spend less time in positive grooming interactions, in part because of the

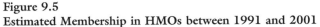

**Figure 9.5**
**Estimated Membership in HMOs between 1991 and 2001**

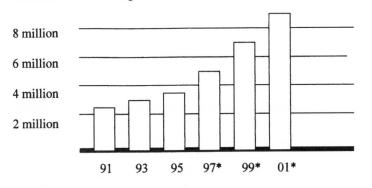

8 million

6 million

4 million

2 million

91    93    95    97*    99*    01*

\* = projected.

dispersion of desired grooming partners. And the positive effects of social ostracism are reduced significantly as a motivating factor for group-enhancing behavior. As quality declines, adversarial relationships increase. Those providers that oppose the decline in quality will conflict with group members who tolerate or condone diminished quality. Dissatisfied patients will complain and some will initiate lawsuits and seek other providers. Some will just give up.

As we mentioned early in this chapter, current projections suggest that there is no immediate end in sight to the trend of healthcare groups increasing in size. One can hardly read the daily newspaper without finding news of another merger of healthcare companies. Big business is not the only culprit, however. Patients of certain ages are also making their mark on bigness. Figure 9.5 provides an example.[4]

Figure 9.5 depicts the number of new seniors that have joined or are projected to join (\* = projected) Medicare managed care plans in the United States from 1991 through 2001. The reasons for these increases are multiple. Polling results from elderly persons who are shifting to Medicare managed care plans indicate that 47% made their decision on the basis of the costs and benefits of available plans, 12% did so on the basis of the providers in the plan, 10% changed because of the advice of friends and relatives, 9% changed because plans were employer or union offered, and 9% changed because of marketing efforts by the plans. Of those that join Medicare managed care plans, approximately 13% do not renew their membership each year.

Looked at from either near or far, the findings in Figure 9.5 point to both the absolute costs of healthcare and cost/benefit ratios as important factors influencing the way patients make healthcare decisions. There is no denying the importance of these variables. The costs of healthcare and cost/

benefit ratios have been central topics in healthcare for at least a decade and a half. Healthcare requires providers, space, and equipment. Providers require salaries. Space, equipment, and salaries require that monies come from somewhere. And so on. So, why are we raising these issues? We are doing so because economic factors are increasingly taking precedence over other factors when healthcare decisions are made. Our point is not that the economics of healthcare is unimportant, but rather that if economic thinking dominates attempts to solve our healthcare conundrum, our solutions will be unsuccessful. Individual and group human nature need to be part of the equation.[5]

Before bringing this chapter to a close, several points deserve to be addressed. First, it is likely that the key architects of future US healthcare plans will object to many of the points we are making. Readers are invited to remain skeptical to their objections. There is literally no evidence that our healthcare systems are improving, or that there are plans on the drawing board that are likely to bring about future improvements. Further, much of what we have said could be incorrectly criticized as a romantic wish to return to the past. Yet we have not once suggested this. We have, however, argued that we can learn from the past and apply these lessons to future healthcare designs.

## CONCLUDING COMMENTS

The main points to be taken from this chapter are that group function, group structure, group size, and quality of care influence one another. Groups that are too small have potential limitations in medicine primarily because they lack the command of knowledge and skills to provide quality care. At the other extreme, groups that are too large are inefficient, divert energies, and do not adequately attend to the details of individual differences. This leaves us with the possibility that medium sized groups may be optimal for 90%+ of our healthcare needs.[6]

## NOTES

1. For an exploration of various social structures, see R. Dunbar and M. Spoors, "Social Networks, Support Cliques, and Kinship," *Human Nature* 6 (1995): 273–290.

2. Such events have corresponding changes in brain physiology as well. See M. T. McGuire and M. J. Raleigh, "Behavioral and Physiological Correlates of Ostracism," *Ethology and Sociobiology* 7 (1986): 39–52.

3. Sometimes ostracism is the alternative to more direct forms of aggression. For a comparison of types of aggression across species, see J. H. Manson and R. W. Wrangham, "Intergroup Aggression in Chimpanzees and Humans," *Current Anthropology* 32 (1991): 369–384.

4. See an article by M. Freudenham in the *New York Times*, 2 August 1997.

5. Sometimes healthcare groups are very vigorous in their competition. See, for example, B. J. Palermo, "The Nastiest Little Fight in Healthcare," *California Medicine* 8(3) (1997): 18–24.

6. For a detailed discussion of the central concepts of this chapter, see M. T. McGuire and A. Troisi, *Darwinian Psychiatry* (New York: Oxford University Press, 1998).

*Part IV*

# Options, Constraints, and Questions

*Chapter 10*

# The Costs, the Benefits, and the Consequences of Group Competition

You ask how I spend my work day. . . . I'll tell you provided you don't reveal my identity. . . . I spend 90% of my time trying to get more clients—that is making more money for the company. . . . For-profit HMOs are like any other business . . . profit is our goal and we will do what we need to do to generate it. . . . Is quality of care important? . . . Of course it is important, but only if we make a profit . . . and if there is a choice, profit comes first. . . . Is my family enrolled in my company? . . . Well . . . yes . . . in part because they can receive services at a reduced cost . . . but if it's anything serious I send them elsewhere. . . . My family is where I draw the line.[1]

Interview with an HMO executive

## INTRODUCTION

Unfortunately for many patients, both public and private debates about US healthcare have failed to move beyond preoccupations with the costs of medical care, who pays for it, and the availability of providers.[2] These are important topics. Yet the moral rhetoric, the political platitudes and maneuvering, and the misinformation that can clutter and misdirect these debates reminds one of the clown searching for his lost keys beneath a street light. A policeman wanders by and joins in the search. After a time, he asks, "Are you sure you lost the keys here?" "I lost them over there," replies the clown, pointing to the dark. "So, why are you looking here?" asks the policeman. "The light's better," replies the clown.

How does the clown's story apply to healthcare? The answer is not difficult to surmise. It is simply easier to add up healthcare costs, argue about who should pay healthcare bills, pass new laws, increase accounting requirements, complain about medical fraud, and devise short-term solutions to pressing healthcare problems than to knuckle down to the hard work of solving issues which, if they remain unsolved, will result in increasing dissatisfaction and reduction in the quality of care.

Chapter 8 argued that our healthcare dilemma would remain unsolved until we take into account basic features of human nature. Cooperation among healthcare players and patients was singled out as a necessary condition for improving existing systems. Chapter 9 focused on group characteristics that can facilitate or impede achieving within-group cooperation, the efficient communication of information, and improvement of healthcare quality. Group size turned out to be a key variable. Groups that are too small have limited capacities to deal with the normal array of medical problems. Groups that are too large develop structures and spawn subgroups that work against cooperation, clear and precise communication, and efficient internal monitoring. We argued that medium size groups, essentially groups not having more than 160 members, have the opportunity of achieving the degree of cooperation and communication efficiency that could ratchet up the quality of healthcare while ratcheting down its costs. Still, size—any size!—is no guarantee that group members will cooperate. Other issues are involved.

This chapter is about large groups and competition within and between them. Such competition has costs. It causes waste. And it diverts efforts to achieve quality and sensible resolutions to healthcare problems. We are talking primarily about the roles of business and government in our current healthcare systems.[3] Like it or not, large groups are now the major players in our healthcare system. Some general points about competition, hierarchy, and assembly-line healthcare will be discussed first. We then turn to look at the healthcare marketplace, technology and assembly-line healthcare, the consequences of competition among large players, and how patients can get lost when marketplace survival takes precedence over patient care.[4] The final sections of the chapter return to a familiar theme, government and healthcare fraud.

## COMPETITION

Competition means that two or more groups compete for the same resources. Applied to nongovernment healthcare organizations, this is usually competition for clients. Clients may be either actual or potential patients. Either way, what is critical is that they have the means to pay for their care or that they have attributes (e.g., age, a recognized disability) which assure that another source such as Medicare, Medicaid, or an insurance company will pay when medical care is provided.

Groups compete for resources for a variety of obvious reasons—financial profit, market power, social influence, prestige, and longevity. Yet there is a more fundamental driving force underlying competition. Individuals, both alone and as group members, engage in competitive activities because they believe that such behavior increases their chances of fulfilling biological goals. Prestige, influence, power, and financial profit are means that can facilitate kin investment, increase the probability of survival, influence reproductive frequency and timing, and affect reciprocal relationships.[5]

On balance, there is probably more to be said for the principle of competition than against it. Numerous studies affirm that both individual and social benefits can accrue when two or more groups compete in the marketplace. Increased productivity, increased product quality, reduced costs, increased profits, and advances in knowledge (research and development) are examples. In instances where benefits develop, there is usually a characteristic set of behaviors. The energy of group members is channeled toward specific goals. Members sense they have a purpose and they work efficiently. And members use their special skills in ways that benefit themselves as well as the group as a whole—a win-win situation for the group, and possibly also for those who interact with the group.

There are also studies affirming another side to competition. These document decreased productivity because of inefficient channeling of energy and creativity, increased costs due to within- and cross-group competition, reduction of quality in favor of excessive profit taking, and fraud. The details of many of these consequences are familiar. Physician groups set up facilities to seize the revenues that are normally funneled to hospitals. Hospitals that for years co-existed peacefully in the same city turn into bitter rivals in their efforts to fill their beds, cut costs, and boost revenues. Some institutions unnecessarily glut local areas with the latest technical equipment in order to attract patients and doctors. New treatments such as laser eye surgery are put in place without adequate research to assess their value or sufficient educational requirements for those providers who offer such treatment. Literally any physician can buy or rent the equipment to carry out these procedures and it is up to patients to ensure that they are not harmed. Unsafe drugs with undesirable health consequences enter the marketplace because the public clamors for them and drug companies are willing to distribute them. The recent history of weight-reducing drugs is an example.[6,7,8] Patients are aware of many of these points and, not surprisingly, increasing numbers of patients have become distrustful of traditional providers and have found a haven in alternative medicine (e.g., acupuncture).

In short, it is the means by which competition is conducted and its outcomes that are important, not the fact that competition takes place.[9,10] Like our desire to survive, competition is part of our nature and particularly so when desirable outcomes are involved. Our proclivities to act competitively are not going to disappear. Given this fact, our most reasonable option is to use competition to the advantage of the healthcare systems we develop. To do so is a nontrivial task, which we address in Chapter 11.

## HIERARCHIES

Hierarchies are systems of social rules, responsibilities, and resource access entitlements that are acknowledged by members of a group. In all groups of two or more individuals, there are some differences in both available resources and resource entitlements. It is these differences that hierarchies are in part designed to administer, defend, and perpetuate, and which often fuel competitive behavior over one's place in a hierarchy.[11]

There are a host of reasons offered for hierarchies. Examples include specifying work responsibilities and resource entitlements of group members, establishing divisions of labor, constraining or positively directing within-group competition, minimizing the adverse effects of free riders, enhancing capacities to compete with other groups, increasing productivity, specifying communication channels, and improving product quality. The list is reasonable if not laudable. There are, however, major underlying problems.

Setting up hierarchies is tantamount to devising and implementing rules applicable to persons at different levels in a multiperson system. This often makes sense from a business perspective. Persons at different positions in hierarchies have different work responsibilities. If a hierarchy is going to work efficiently, it is essential to define these responsibilities and to educate and monitor individuals to assure that they are doing their jobs well. Similar points apply to information. Frequent meetings are required to assure that individuals are properly informed about what they need to know, how to use their knowledge, and so forth.[12]

Such activities do not take place in a vacuum. Time and energy costs are involved for those who design, perpetuate, and participate in even the most efficient of hierarchies. In addition, human factors inevitably come into play, and they often work against both the efficiency and aims of hierarchical systems. Hierarchy members spend considerable time trying to determine if others are receiving special treatment. They compete with each other for advancement and increased access to resources. In the process they often divert resources to assure their own success and longevity rather than to enhance the goals of the group. Human time and energy as well as resource costs are involved in each of these activities.[13,14,15]

Much of what we have said thus far is common knowledge. Thus, it is reasonable to inquire into the costs of hierarchies and within-group competition. There are no well-documented answers to this question and the costs will differ from group to group. Yet those figures that have been published are informative. They reveal, for example, that approximately 40% of every dollar paid to large healthcare players, which for this discussion means insurance companies and HMOs, goes to what typically are called administrative costs. Administrative costs cover such items as paying people to administer claims, to hire personnel, to advertise, to communicate with the outside world, and to compete with other providers in the marketplace. Administrative costs also cover executives' salaries, shareholders' profits, and special entitlements. What they do not cover is hands-on healthcare. Turned upside down, 40% means that only 60% of each healthcare dollar is available for patient care. (While federal and state governments generally do not have stockholders or make a profit, a reasonable assumption is that their administrative costs exceed 40%.) This is far from efficient allocation or use of funds. It is all the more inefficient when it is recognized that there are additional administrative costs at the hands-on treatment level.

## TECHNOLOGY AND ASSEMBLY-LINE HEALTHCARE

In principle, it would be reasonable to expect that much of the administrative cost of healthcare could be reduced through technological advances and assembly-line care delivery. Large companies like Ford and General Motors exist and make profits while employing thousands of persons. Much of their longevity is due to two facts: technological advances reduce many of the costs of production (though not necessarily of materials) and the tasks involved in production can be effectively separated so that efficient assembly-line techniques can be utilized.[16]

The part played by technology in medicine is particularly interesting and has two facets. One has to do with technologies that improve diagnostic capacities and treatment options. PET and MRI have already been mentioned. EKG machines, computers that tell brain surgeons where to look for lesions, electronic systems that monitor heart rate, blood pressure, and breathing rate, and dialysis machines are other examples. For the most part, providers have quickly accepted these technological advances and put them to good use, but with a rise in costs of healthcare that was discussed earlier. In effect, competition between groups—everyone needs an MRI machine— and oversight authorities demand such machines, hence the rise in costs.

The second facet has to do with the collection, organization, and dissemination of clinically relevant information such as patients' histories, disease intervention strategies, and the details of treatment responses. Some of these activities have been streamlined by technological advances such as the use of flow charts and computer programs designed to manage diverse types of information, but the degree of progress lags far behind machines that carry out their work on their own.

Why is it that providers who may be perfectly familiar with all types of technologies still write medical records, still call laboratories for test results, and still spend more time talking with each other than using e-mail? There is no mystery here. Much of the important information that is relevant to patient care is carried in the minds of providers. It is counterproductive to try to record much of this information into even the most user-friendly and efficient computers. Healthcare, and especially quality healthcare, is far too complex, has far too many intangibles, and is far too contingent on changing conditions for computers to help with a large percentage of important clinical work.[17]

Facets of healthcare systems can use assembly-line techniques and at the same time improve quality of care and contain costs. Labor can be divided so that there are specialists to draw blood, administer EKGs, prepare persons for surgery, immunize children, and analyze the chemical makeup of tissue samples. Much of this already occurs. Yet this approach holds up only so far. When we get down to diagnosis and treatment, other issues crop up. Unlike automobiles, no two patients are ever quite the same, and because they are not, assembly-line medicine can result in as much harm as help. For any healthcare system, the people who enter the system each day will differ. The desired products (optimal diagnosis and treatment) perhaps can be partially specified in advance. But the means by which optimal treatment is achieved will differ from patient to patient. Success is contingent on examining the patients making an accurate diagnosis, understanding the patient's mental state, and selecting an appropriate, patient-relevant treatment option. Recently, dissatisfaction with assembly-line medicine has become so great among many providers that they have decoupled themselves from HMOs and attempted to reestablish patient-oriented practices.[18]

To digress for a moment, in the process of preparing this book one of the authors interviewed a number of medical administrators. The aim of these interviews was to find out their thoughts about healthcare delivery in the year 2010. Not unexpectedly, there was a range of responses. However, a common theme was apparent in over 80% of the interviews. Healthcare in 2010 will be "technologized" and have many of the characteristics of the assembly line. Patients will enter a system. They will be given a set of routine examinations, tested in a variety of ways, and so forth. These events will occur long before patients see a professional provider, and the information they provide will be assembled in a highly condensed form much like shorthand. The provider will review the assembled material, see the patient for perhaps seven minutes and, in most instances, order prescriptions by speaking into a voice activated computer, which will communicate the information to the pharmacy. As the patient leaves the provider's office, he will be handed a paper bag containing his medications and instructions about the use of the medications. Should the patient want to talk further about his medical condition, he will be directed to a special group of medical interpreters who will offer translations of the provider's thoughts and, within limits, listen to patients' concerns. Much as we may hope that the medical year 2010 never arrives, the speculations of these administrators should not be underestimated. Given the current course of US healthcare, assembly-line medicine will have a significant influence on tomorrow's practice.[19]

The motivations and capacities to deliver quality healthcare are special capacities. Not all individuals have these qualities. More important, these capacities do not readily fit into convenient marketplace categories, in much the same way that writings of poets and musical scores of composers often do not readily fit into the marketplace. To the degree that the assembly-line mentality dominates healthcare, its most talented providers will be constrained. Readers should ask themselves whether they want to be a number in a medical assembly line, or if they want to donate approximately 40% of their healthcare dollar to administrators who have little to do with the hands-on features of healthcare, and if they think that the medical care that will be provided in the future will be optimal.

The upshot of the preceding points is that technological advances are highly worthwhile in some areas of healthcare, yet only tangentially so in other areas. The fact that many of the key hands-on features of healthcare have not been significantly improved by modern technology speaks to a point that we have stressed repeatedly: When one deals with individual differences there are limits to the degree to which technology and assembly-line approaches can help. These points have yet to dawn on many of the architects of tomorrow's medicine. Nevertheless, given current blueprints, if the direction of things does not change, most of those reading this book can expect to experience assembly-line medicine—2010 is not that far away.

## THE MARKETPLACE AND GROUP COMPETITION

This brings us to the marketplace and cross-group competition. There are well-known costs that accrue from entering the marketplace, such as the costs of product research and development, purchasing materials, manufacturing, advertising, and hiring employees. There is, however, another critically important factor that operates in the marketplace, and it involves the costs of competition. As noted, individual HMOs and insurance companies do not operate as if they are the only players in the healthcare world. They compete with each other for many of the same resources and patients.[20] When they do, operational costs rise because of the time and effort required to compete. Figure 10.1 illustrates this point.

Figure 10.1 depicts the estimated total amount of resources devoted to marketplace competition by a single competitor when it is competing with other groups for the same resources. The numbers on the horizontal axis should be taken as approximations. One to five groups signify a small number of competitors in the marketplace. Six to fifteen groups signify a larger number of competitors and that competition is more intense. Greater than 20 groups signify that competition is extremely intense, that the fortunes of

**Figure 10.1**
**Estimated Changes in Resource Allocation as a Function of the Number of Competitors in the Marketplace**

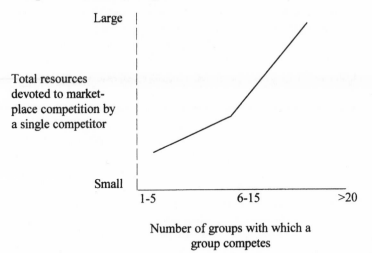

Number of groups with which a
group competes

*Source:* Authors.

competitors are uncertain, and that if profits are to be made, cost control and expense cutting are likely.[21]

As the number of groups in competition increases, a point is reached where there is a rapid increase in the associated costs. A number of factors are responsible. One is that more time is spent in monitoring the activities of competitors. Another is the time and effort spent in internal adjustments in order to compete successfully. Both procedural and informational adjustments are relevant here. Procedural adjustments deal with new rules, such as who reports to whom and who is responsible for what. Informational adjustments deal with the dissemination of information, who will control it, who will transmit it, who will receive it, and who can act on it.

Where a competitor is located in Figure 10.1 will influence its capacities to provide quality services. For example, one recent study asked physicians to rate three different plans from the perspective of whether or not they would recommend the plan for their families. Sixty-four percent said they would recommend Plan A, 24% said they would recommend Plan B, and 92% would recommend Plan C. The 92% figure is encouraging, but such a high number appears relatively infrequently. Evaluations of physician provider groups by patients point to a different set of issues. In one study, less than 80% of patients were satisfied with the overall quality of their care, only 60% felt that the quality of their care was adequate, less than 60% found it easy to get care or referrals, less than 60% felt that doctors had acceptable communication skills, and less than 30% believed that they were receiving preventive care counseling. The evaluations are not much better with physician groups. For example, in one study, 27 medical groups were surveyed. Consumers, or patients, gave the groups an overall score of 64 on a scale of 100 for quality of care, a score 59 for the ease of getting care and specialist referrals, and a score of 62 for doctors' communication skills. (Although there are exceptions, generally the larger the plan the lower the rating.)

It might be hoped that technological advances such as e-mail and person-to-person video will reduce the time and effort spent in transmitting information, altering arrangements within groups, and so forth. However, this view ignores several obvious points about human nature. People like face-to-face communication and the grooming that goes with it—homeostasis is important. E-mail simply is not fully effective when it comes to grooming. Furthermore, do not expect things to change much when we can sit at our computer monitors and see the person with whom we are communicating. We are social animals and touching, sitting next to, smelling, and nonverbal signaling count. Despite thousands of pounds of documents, thousands of e-mail transmissions, and hundreds of videos dealing with rules and adjustments, most of the important information in any business is still communicated by word of mouth. Moreover, sending e-mail, developing videos, and writing and editing manuals requires time and energy. Even the most detailed manuals specifying how one should behave are seldom so clear and so all-inclusive that considerable amplification via face-to-face discussion is not required.[22,23]

In effect, because of cross-group competition, the costs of doing business increase. If so, costs need to be reduced somewhere else. As noted, too often the reductions occur in the number of available healthcare providers and in a like reduction of available procedures. When considerations of cost containment and competition begin to dominate healthcare, healthcare loses its sensitivity and responsivity. "Lean and mean" is fine when running the marathon, but it is not what is needed for optimal healthcare.[24]

## COST CUTTING AND PROFIT TAKING

Costs are relevant to the preceding points. Unlike the assembly lines of automobile companies where new technology can reduce costs and improve product quality, many of the technological advances in medicine such as PET, MRI, DNA typing, complex surgeries, and dialysis significantly increase the costs of diagnosis and treatment. Chemicals need to be purchased. MRI machines need to be maintained. Someone needs to collect blood and administer dialysis. Operating rooms need to be scrubbed and decontaminated. These are expensive activities and their costs find their ways into hospital charges and provider bills. As they do, one of four things happens. Patients are asked to pay more. The government steps in to pay a percentage of the bills. Medical bills do not get paid. Or HMOs and insurance companies respond by trying to contain costs through limiting services.[25] It is cost containment and profit taking that are the topics of this section.

Insurance companies and HMOs want to survive. With a few exceptions, such as nonprofit healthcare insurance companies like Blue Shield, they want to make a profit—what else is business about? Even "nonprofit" insurance companies are influenced by the same incentives to increase operating margins and cash flow. Because they want to survive, they will do what is necessary to assure survival. Cutting costs in a competitive marketplace is one of the time-honored ways to remain competitive and increase the chances of survival. Numerous cost-cutting methods have been tried. Introducing deductibles on medical costs is one. This simply amounts to charging patients more for their healthcare. Reducing the length of hospital stays is another. In many instances, shortened stays have not appreciably reduced the quality of care. Thus, within limits, the reduction of services does not necessarily imply that quality of care will decline, although even here it is necessary to examine the costs of medical care provided by nonprofessionals such as relatives once one leaves the hospital. Turning over diagnostic and therapeutic decisions to nonprofessional personnel is yet another cost-cutting mechanism. This practice has its obvious limitations. And subcontracting specific procedures (e.g., autopsies) is still another example of short-term cost-cutting efforts. As business-wise as these efforts may appear to be, they often turn out to have the opposite effects from those that were originally intended, particularly when cost cutting leads to errors in diagnosis, suboptimal treatments, and increases in hospital readmission rates.

More perverse ways of containing costs are to reduce either the frequency with which costly medical procedures are performed or the number of available healthcare providers. It is here that competition and hierarchy return to the discussion. Consider the following example. A healthcare insurance company or an HMO sets up a system that attempts to contain the costs of healthcare among its subscribers. When the short-term options have been exploited, the one remaining alternative is to reduce the frequency with which healthcare services are provided to clients. This translates to a reduction in the use of procedures, the availability of healthcare providers, or both.

How HMOs and insurance companies go about deciding which procedures should be targeted for reduced availability differs. Yet, in principle, the underlying processes and the results are the same. First, someone in the company decides that a medical procedure or service is provided more often than someone (from a business perspective) thinks is necessary. Next, there is an examination of the use of the procedure or service and its possible medical effectiveness. For some inexpensive procedures such as taking temperatures or measuring blood pressure, there is very little debate. It is when procedures are expensive that debate begins. Third, a "task force" decides on a set of rules for the use of the procedures. Fourth, someone writes the set of rules. Fifth, the rules are transmitted to subscribers (patients), health-care providers that work with the HMO or the insurance company, and to those persons within the company (gatekeepers) who will decide whether or not a procedure or service can or cannot be used.

Once these steps have been taken, use of a procedure requires HMO or insurance company approval, otherwise the costs of the procedure or service will be denied. In effect, gatekeepers determine if a procedure will be used. Again, such actions may make sense from a business standpoint. However, from a quality-of-care standpoint they often backfire. Gatekeepers are at the very bottom of the HMO and insurance company hierarchies. Their capacity to make decisions is limited by a set of rules they must follow or lose their jobs. They are often uninformed about the reasons for the rules. They frequently know very little about medicine. If rules need to be overridden, supervisors must be contacted. From the standpoint of the healthcare provider and the patient he or she is treating, hours, sometimes days, are spent dealing with gatekeepers, and even then, an essential procedure may be denied. One outcome of these events is that the costs of doing business are transferred from insurance companies and HMOs to providers and patients. Further, the total costs of medical care may increase. Either way, the quality of care declines.

Let us be perfectly clear about numbers in medicine. It is all well and good to apply numbers to medical procedures such as one of every 60 women who receive a mammogram will have some form of cancer. The problem with numbers, however, is that they do not apply at the individual level. If a patient happens to be the one female in 60 who has early mammary cancer, she will want it detected, even though number-sensitive providers may not find it cost-effective to provide such examinations.

The reduction of healthcare providers works in similar ways. Providers such as doctors, nurses, and laboratory assistants are usually highly educated, extensively trained, and costly. An HMO that removes a physician from its roles can save as much as $300,000 per year when salaries, employment benefits, and support personnel are woven into the cost-saving equation. The temptation to decrease the number of costly personnel is very attractive from the business perspective, and no doubt this is why individual providers are often given their walking papers.[26,27]

When gatekeepers go to work and provider numbers are reduced, the events that follow are all too familiar. Dozens of telephone calls and long waits become a fact of life if one wishes to obtain a medical appointment. Sometimes phones are not answered. Delays in decisions about treatments become commonplace. Patients become anxious and angry. Further, there is no discernable bottom line to these intrusions into quality. Daily, an increasing number of procedures need to be authorized and daily it takes longer to contact one's healthcare provider. As the gates get higher and the number of providers gets lower, do the top and middle managers lose their jobs? Seldom. Do companies that engage in cost cutting increase their profits? Often. Are there more providers to care for clients in a more timely and expert way? Rarely. Yet the costs of healthcare do not seem to decrease and the 35% to 40% figures for administrative costs persist despite technological advances and attempts to introduce assembly-line techniques.

When companies become preoccupied with profits and cost cutting, concerns about quality tend to disappear. What is forgotten is that quality medicine is customized medicine. Quality medicine has high and unavoidable interaction costs. For example, we estimate that the average front-line healthcare provider working for a large group spends approximately 30–40% of his or her time dealing directly with patients. The remaining time is spent in within-group and cross-group activities. We also estimate that 70% interaction time is required to achieve consistently high-quality delivery of care for the same number of patients. When the percentage drops below 70%, medical errors increase because healthcare professionals have less time to spend with patients, less time to assimilate new knowledge, and their motivation to produce quality care declines. In turn, patient dissatisfaction increases. When it does, more legislation is sought, more lawsuits are initiated, and more money is spent on activities that are remote from the original purpose of healthcare systems. It follows that looking only to the marketplace to solve the healthcare problems in the United States may be looking in the wrong place.

## COMPETITION AND FRAUD

It is somewhere in the preceding picture that fraud becomes attractive. Medical fraud is not a trivial issue—it is estimated to be at least a $100-billion a year business and it is often the quick road to profit. The reason hot dog vendors are rarely accused of fraud is because there is a clear relationship between the product purchased and its cost. A dollar changes hands as does a hot dog. It is an easy give-and-take system to understand. However, in complex systems with their sophisticated accounting practices and with low probability that they will be audited, simple and transparent exchanges seldom occur.[28]

How does medical fraud work? The principle is straightforward. A provider, say a doctor, submits a claim for treatment that he or she has not provided. If the claim is submitted to an insurance company or the government, it will usually be paid unless there is some reason to disallow it. Disallowances usually require investigations, which means time and money and thus constraints on the number of investigations that are undertaken. When bills are unlikely to be audited, fraudulent behavior becomes attractive. HMOs engage in the same behavior. They just play on a larger scale and use more sophisticated methods, such as altering billing and accounting practices. Unfortunately, despite numerous investigations, and despite the amount of suspected fraud, few convictions follow. At times, irritated insiders blow the whistle. There are constraints working against such behavior, however. To blow the whistle on one's colleagues is to invite retaliation and endanger one's future employment, a point underscored by the recent congressional hearings dealing with the Internal Revenue Service (IRS). Whistleblowers appeared at the hearing wearing bags over their heads and using voice modulators.[29]

## GOVERNMENT INTERVENTIONS

When fraud occurs in the marketplace and there are enough complaints, sometimes someone in government moves to action. President Clinton announced a plan to investigate surging Medicare fraud. As this chapter is being written, his concern is with home healthcare, which accounts for a rapidly growing percentage of the fraudulent activity. Federal investigations will start. Grand juries will be formed. Investigative squads will be organized and sent into the public and private domain. And so forth.

Interactions between HMOs, insurance companies, and the government generally make healthcare more costly and divisive.[30] In the healthcare field, the intrusion of government usually means the introduction of rules and procedures that are difficult to understand, let alone to follow. Eventually, however, and despite its best intentions, government often loses control of its efforts to achieve specific goals.[31]

Signs of loss of control are everywhere. Diagnostic and treatment services are rationed. Government proposals designed to increase responsibilities of provider organizations and limit their abuses are put forth and enacted into law. More dollars are allocated to areas that are thought to be insufficiently funded. New federal panels are developed to assess problems. Government projections of its ability to pay for Medicare point to a dismal future— $2,000,000,000,000 (2 trillion) is the projected medical cost for the United States in the year 2007.[32] HMOs continue their revolving door policy and frequently abandon the poor after they have taken their dollars. The private medical market continues to atrophy. Academic healthcare centers come under increasing attack. Employers switch healthcare plans because of cost differences, thereby decreasing continuity of care. Accountability requirements increase. And new audit groups spring up.

Literally no player in the medical field is exempt from contributing to the current chaos. Patients often make excessive demands and have unrealistic expectations of medical services. Government patches here and there without addressing fundamental issues. HMOs and insurance companies continue to pursue profit despite the consequences. Hospitals continue to pursue the strategy of being at once public and private institutions, charities and businesses, welfare institutions and icons of US science. No one wants to change.[33]

When control is lost, political solutions are usually sought, and far too frequently this means that the proposed solutions will lack coherence and serve more as Band Aids than as means of bringing about needed improvements to healthcare. For example, as of this writing, 50 bills have passed the California Legislative Assembly and 30 more are pending in the California Senate. Bills take many forms: for example, HMOs can't dismiss a doctor without arbitration; HMO personnel making medical decisions must be licensed physicians; authority for the management of HMOs should be transferred to a special state unit; minimum hospital stays should be permitted after certain types of medical procedures and childbirth; and HMOs can not merge unless the state approves. Examples of federal bills include: a shift in Medicare dollars away from the urban HMOs to rural HMOs; the development of interstate healthcare pools; the reduction of Medicare payments; and increasing the age when Medicare payments start while lowering the age at which individuals can "buy into" Medicare.[34,35,36]

## WHERE ARE THE PATIENTS?

Where are the patients in all of this? The answer is that they are in one of two places. First, they remain important as sources of revenue and minimal expenses. Thus, there is some need for healthcare providers and healthcare payers to pay attention to them. Second, they are the recipients of cost cuts and healthcare disorganization. In such circumstances, it might be expected that patients would revolt, and in some cases, they have. Recently elderly Californians demonstrated against the confusion inherent in their healthcare systems, the services they are being denied and the quality of their care. However, the effectiveness of occasional protests in changing the existing healthcare system is limited. Moreover, even if patients banded together, understanding the many facets of the healthcare system is likely to be beyond both their interest and knowledge.[37]

## CONCLUDING COMMENTS

This chapter has been about some of the unfortunate consequences that large organizations, marketplace competition, and government can bring to healthcare. It seems doubtful to us that these consequences will disappear even if all players acted on their best behavior. There are simply too many factors involved that work against such an outcome. Big business and government are complex systems and much as they might try, there are constraints on their abilities to achieve certain objectives. Other solutions are needed to whip our healthcare into the shape it ought to be.

## NOTES

1. For an inside story of the profit-driven life in modern healthcare, see L. Lagnado, *Wall Street Journal*, 30 May 1997.

2. President Clinton's Health Panel is likely to propose two entities, one public and one private, to set healthcare goals and standards. See L. McGinley, *Wall Street Journal*, 12 March 1998.

3. Some are of the opinion that there is atrophy in the private medical market and that the government should contribute to an infrastructure that can lead to universal coverage. See B. M. Smith, "Trends in Health Care Coverage and Financing their Implications for Policy," *New England Journal of Medicine*, 2 October 1997.

4. HMOs increasingly control where patients are treated, and only large hospital groups have the power to contract with them on a relatively equal basis. The strategy of the Catholic hospitals has been based on the idea that growth may be a matter of survival. See M. Langley, in *Wall Street Journal*, 7 January 1998, which gives insight into a Catholic hospital chain and its financial reserves.

5. Sometimes competition for resources can cause conflict between hospitals and physicians. See, for example, an article by M. Langley in the *Wall Street Journal*, 25 November 1997.

6. Lawyers are preparing for a deluge of diet drug ("Fen-Phen") lawsuits. An interesting feature of the removal of Redux and Pondimin from the market was the speed with which lawyers actively entered the market. See L. Johannes and A. Schmitt, *Wall Street Journal*, 17 September 1997.

7. America Home Products, which has sold the diet drugs domestically, is attempting to get information on reports of heart valve problems. See L. Johannes, *Wall Street Journal*, 1 October 1997.

8. The diet drug Fen-Phen has been removed from the market following information suggesting that it may cause heart valve problems. See the report of M. Cimons, *Los Angeles Times*, 16 September 1997.

9. Physicians are increasingly operating outside the HMO structure because of their view that the quality of care has been compromised. See D. Olmos, "Doctors Seek 'Un-Managed' Client Base," *Los Angeles Times*, 9 April 1998.

10. The Congressional Budget Office estimates that by 2007 the United States will be spending over $2 trillion on healthcare annually and that 53% of these expenditures will be government dollars. See E. Ginzberg and M. Ostow, *New England Journal of Medicine*, 31 July 1997.

11. The variety of healthcare services makes any system of accountability difficult. See H. Larkin, "Market, Legal Pressures Push Health System Accountability, But Is It Enough?" *Advances* 1 (1998): 1–2.

12. Healthcare plans themselves may be thought of as having a hierarchy, at least as judged by physicians. See, for example, S. J. Borowsky et al., "Are All Health Plans Created Equal? The Physician's View," *Journal of the American Medical Association* 278 (1997): 917–921.

13. Problems with hierarchy tend to become most visible at the time that a merger is being considered. Consider an article by R. Rundle, "Home-Health Rivals Try Merger of Equals, Get Merger from Hell," *Wall Street Journal*, 7 April 1998. Two large HMOs tried to combine but could not work out the power-related details, and now both suffer.

14. Academic medical centers also suffer problems of hierarchy when they try to cooperate or merge. See an article by L. Lagnado in the *Wall Street Journal*, 21 March 1997. New York University and Sinai Medical Centers tried for eight months to merge and finally were unable to find an appropriate way to combine the two hospitals. The doctors, aware that merging would mean reducing staff and positions of power, clashed over whose school and hospital were better, who would wield how much authority, where classes would be held, and even how the minutes of the merger meetings would be kept.

15. Problems with hierarchy also exist within separate divisions of the same corporation. L. Scism and S. Paltrow, *Wall Street Journal*, 7 August 1997, document how Prudential's auditors gave early warnings about sales abuses and how management didn't listen. There is a moral in the Prudential story addressing the assumption that auditors provide us with a safe world.

16. Assembly lines are not always compatible with medical procedures. See, for example, G. Jaffe, "Need an Autopsy?" *Wall Street Journal*, 2 July 1997, in which we see how hospitals have abandoned autopsies and turned them over to small businesses. How much important medical information may be lost is not yet known.

17. Communication between professionals remains problematic, whether or not there is attempted computer enhancement. See H. R. Bernard, P. D. Killworth, and L. Sailer, "Information Accuracy in Social-Network Data: V. An Experimental Attempt to Predict Actual Communication from Recall Data," *Social Science Research* 11 (1982): 30–66. The authors provide compelling evidence that what people say about their communications bears no resemblance to their behavior.

18. Considerable tension exists between those who believe that physicians should become more business-oriented and those who believe they should retain a patient-centered attitude. See an article by S. Roan in the *Wall Street Journal*, 16 June 1997, in which the author discusses the recommendations of a University of California commission that has urged medical schools to emphasize business skills and clinic experience to meet the demands of managed care.

19. The quest for human uniformity never sleeps. See, for example, K. Dowling, "Clinton Care: Feds Replace the Family," *Los Angeles Times*, 8 March 1998, in which the author outlines some of the implications of the Clinton view towards the American people, including that mothers are obsolete, cradle-to-grave government is desirable, and standardized day care is the answer for many of the problems of youth.

20. One of the chief ways HMOs compete is in the critical area of patient selection and extrusion. See R. Morgan and colleagues, "The Medicare Revolving Door—The Healthy Go In and the Sick Go Out," *New England Journal of Medicine*, 17 July 1997, in which the authors present data showing marked selection biases with respect to HMO enrollment and disenrollment.

21. Competition among many HMOs tends to cause them to promise more than they can deliver. See G. Anders and R. Winslow, *Wall Street Journal*, 22 December 1997, in which the authors document in detail how the HMO business has turned

sour and how many HMO woes are a consequence of conflicting demands of the American public. Many patients expect lower costs as well as special treatment.

22. See T. Bodenheimer and K. Sullivan, "How Large Employers Are Shaping the Health Care Marketplace," *New England Journal of Medicine*, 2 April 1998. Because employers are sensitive to price differences they often switch from one care system to another to save money. One effect is that physician–patient relationships are disrupted.

23. See M. Freudenheim, *New York Times*, 2 August 1997, in which the author reviews how seniors are moving to managed care plans and the reasons for their doing so. Cost is the primary consideration regardless of the quality of the plan.

24. One way of being lean (and sometimes mean) is to restrict the budget for prescription drugs. See, for example, L. Johannes, *Wall Street Journal*, 22 May 1997.

25. One of the most effective ways to contain costs is to extrude whole classes patients with lower than average payment. See R. Langreth, "After Seeking Profits from the Poor, Some HMOs Abandon Them," *Wall Street Journal*, 7 April 1998.

26. Organized labor has shown increasing interest in membership drives in the healthcare arena. See, for example, G. Burkins, *Wall Street Journal*, 8 July 1997.

27. Academic professionals have expressed increased interest in union representation as well. See an article by K. Combs in the *Daily Bruin*, 30 September 1997, in which the author documents how healthcare professionals in the University of California system have voted to join a union in order to have a say in the development of healthcare policy.

28. Deception and fraud may intrude anywhere, it seems. E. Tanouye, *Wall Street Journal*, 15 September 1997, explores some of the implications of altered research documents among drug producers.

29. See. T. Lowry, *USA Today*, 8 August 1997, for a discussion of how insiders are increasingly the whistleblowers on healthcare fraud.

30. Bureaucrats tend to minimize the costs that go with regulations. In the *Los Angeles Times*, 17 February 1998, author A. Rubin reviews how Democrats in Congress are attempting to develop tough healthcare plans. Not unexpectedly, opponents are reported to fear increasing costs and an increasing number of lawsuits. The article chronicles some of the problems that develop with the legislative approach to solving medical problems and the contrast between good intentions and actual outcomes.

31. Sometimes it is necessary for government regulators to intervene in a major way by revocation of licenses. See an article by D. Olmos in the *Los Angeles Times*, 3 April 1997, in which the author documents how the Kaiser system is facing the threat of a shutdown in Texas. State officials say they may withdraw the firm's license over problems with patient care and poor financial health.

32. There may be a limit even to the deep pockets of the government. A. Sharpe reports in the *Wall Street Journal*, 1 May 1997, how doctors and hospitals chase poor pregnant women and lucrative reimbursements. As a result, Medicaid, the federal and state program that funds healthcare for much of the nation's poor, has emerged as the industry's generous uncle.

33. Interesting alliances are sometimes made. See, for example, D. Blumenthal et al., "The Social Missions of Academic Health Centers," *New England Journal of Medicine*, 22 November 1997. The authors argue for a strong pro-government view of academic centers and suggest that such centers must undergo major changes if they wish to retain their special position.

34. Demographic changes are often not factored into analysis in a timely way. See M. Angell, "Fixing Medicare," *New England Journal of Medicine*, 17 July 1997, in which the author argues that Medicare will be inadequate when the baby boomers reach retirement age and that alternatives should be considered soon.

35. Rationing is often said to be an essential feature of any rational system. See T. Bodenheimer, MD, "The Oregon Health Plan—Lessons for the Nation," *New England Journal of Medicine*, 28 August 1997, in which the author outlines the pros and cons of the Oregon Health Plan, which is the first serious attempt by a state to ration healthcare.

36. Care of special populations such as children have become an increasing political concern. See P. Newacheck, et al., "Health Insurance and Access to Primary Care for Children," *New England Journal of Medicine*, 19 February 1998, in which the authors argue that the health insurance program enacted as part of the Balanced Budget Act of 1997 may improve access to the use of primary care by children.

37. Still, the impulse to reform through law and regulation will be a part of our concerns for a long time. See an article by M. Vanzi and C. Ingram in the *Los Angeles Times*, 17 June 1997, in which the authors document how California state legislators have launched an onslaught of HMO reform efforts. All deal with limiting HMO options.

*Chapter 11*

# Viable Healthcare Options

---

It's crazy . . . the rules change so often I can't keep track of them. . . .
I know we're making mistakes and breaking laws or rules, but which
ones—who knows? . . . I've added fifteen employees in the last two years
simply to keep us up with the rules. . . . Fifteen employees is an 80%
increase in my work force. . . . Still, we are behind and we are more
confused than five years ago. . . . I'd be out of here in a minute if I didn't
have four mouths to feed.

> Interview with the billing department
> manager at a large urban hospital

## INTRODUCTION

Sickness and disease are not illusions. They are part of nature. They are not
going to go away. They need to be diagnosed and treated now and in the
future.

Workplace injuries occur at a rate of 12 to 13 million per year, and the
rate varies little from year to year.[1] Genes—they too are not going to go
away—play a contributing role in more than 50% of chronic diseases. As the
number of elderly persons increases yearly, the number of persons with
chronic diseases also increases.[2] New forms of viruses and bacteria make their
debut each autumn and spring, meaning that tomorrow's disease picture
will not be the same as today's. Twenty years ago no one would have predicted that AIDS would be a worldwide epidemic or that tuberculosis would
be again on the rise. There is no sense in leaving planning for tomorrow
until tomorrow. Now is the better choice.

This chapter is about essential principles that apply to healthcare solutions for tomorrow. It is not about fantasies, fads, or hyperbolae that have no anchors in reality. It is not about hopes that the marketplace, when left to its own devices, or government, even in its ideal form, can provide acceptable healthcare solutions. Three decades of marketplace solutions to healthcare have left us with a mixed bag of outcomes, most of which are difficult to defend, and literally none of which is likely to survive in the future. The story with government is much the same. Government's cumbersome and hierarchical structure, as well as its bureaucratic ways of conducting business, means that it will trip nearly every time it takes a step in healthcare.

We begin this chapter with some general comments and a review of points that are critical to include in any system design that aims to achieve quality healthcare. In effect, we address the following question: "If healthcare systems are to provide accessible, predictable, high-quality care, what are the guidelines that will give these goals a chance of becoming a reality?" We then turn to illustrative scenarios. The final part of the chapter addresses possible responses to our recommendations.

## GENERAL POINTS

We have argued that many of the problems that face healthcare in the United States will remain unresolved if healthcare delivery, quality, and cost containment are left to HMOs,[3] insurance companies,[4] or the government.[5,6] Where does this leave us? Our answer is that viable solutions can be found only if healthcare is approached from a new perspective. The essentials of this perspective are that fundamental facts of individual and group human nature must be included in the design and operation of any healthcare system that expects to have longevity, achieve quality, and contain costs. Our emphasis on human nature does not mean that other relevant facts should be excluded or that they are unimportant. Economic facts are as much a part of medicine as medicine is a part of economics. Appointments with patients need to be made, providers need to be well trained and need to update their knowledge, and medical supplies need to be purchased. Each of these activities costs money.

What are these fundamental facts of individual and group human nature? Consider patients first. (1) Patients will act to improve their chances of successful survival, kin investment, reciprocal relationships, and reproduction. (2) They will act to reduce uncertainty. Uncertainty is not limited to specific medical issues, such as diagnosis or the likelihood that a specific treatment will work, although these clearly are associated with uncertainty. It extends to such areas as whether providers will be available to answer the phone, whether today's providers will also be tomorrow's providers, whether there will be adequate medical responses in emergency situations, and whether costs make certain types of healthcare unfeasible.

A different set of facts applies to hands-on providers. (1) Providers will act to improve their own as well as their patients' chances of successful survival, kin investment, and reproduction. They will attempt to reduce uncertainty. They will do a better job if patients cooperate, if providers receive a reasonable income, and if providers have control over their professional decisions. (2) Providers will actively monitor and correct healthcare if the criteria of quality are reasonable and the social consequences for suboptimal quality are apparent.

Yet other facts apply to payers. (1) Patients, when considered as payers, will invest resources to increase their chances of predictable, quality healthcare, provided the costs are reasonable. (2) Patients, again considered as payers, will act to increase the quality of healthcare per unit of investment. (3) Insurance companies and HMOs will act to make a profit from healthcare and, over time, profit will be more important than the services they provide. (4) Government will act to improve healthcare, but its costs will be excessive, healthcare delivery will be unequal, and constraints will be excessively restrictive and insensitive to individual differences.

## INTEGRATION

How do these critical facts get translated into workable healthcare systems? This is a question about function. Efficient function refers to cost-effective ways of achieving the specified goals of healthcare—that is, goals that take into account facts, systems, patients, providers, and payers.

System design must accommodate to the fact that quality healthcare is both time consuming and at times expensive, although it need not be prohibitively expensive. At best, diagnosis, intervention choice, and illness management are mixtures of science and art.[7] If quality is to be achieved, there are limits to the degree to which the human and technical costs of healthcare can be reduced.[8] There will be may diagnostic tests that will be nonrevealing just as there will be many questions asked by clinicians, administrators, CEOs, and government employees that will be nonrevealing.[9]

Patients (both as recipients of services and as payers) as well as providers must be integrated into the design, operation, and monitoring of healthcare systems. In effect, tomorrow's healthcare systems need to shift from either their traditional service-and-pay model or the more recent marketplace and government models to *cooperation-service models*. Recall that the probability of cooperation increases when it is in the best interest of participants to cooperate. To devise systems requiring individuals to act in ways that are inconsistent with their nature, that is in ways that are counter to both their predispositions and reasonable expectations, is to invite noncooperation, distraction, the inefficient use of resources, and frustration. The initial burden of proof that cooperation is possible is a joint opportunity for both patients and providers.

Providers must accept the fact that there is an upper limit to the amount of money they can expect to earn. While physicians receive less than 10% of the healthcare dollar, their contribution to containing costs is important. Likewise, patients must accept the fact that they will have to participate far more than they now do in the design, management, delivery, and assessment of healthcare—every hour a patient contributes to a healthcare system is an hour less that must be purchased. Healthcare insurance companies will have to accept the fact that they are in the wrong business unless they limit their insurance to catastrophic claims. HMOs will have to accept the fact that they cannot be accountable to two masters simultaneously—profit and quality care. Government will have to accept the fact that there are some dilemmas that it can not resolve.

New healthcare systems must be responsive to two critical facts of system design. First, there is no single optimal healthcare system configuration—a pediatric outpatient clinic should be structured and staffed differently than a care facility for the elderly. Second, group size and structure have a significant impact on both resource allocation and quality of care.

For general medical care, groups of providers that are small (< 25 members) are unlikely to provide comprehensive quality healthcare although they may be able to contain costs. There is simply too much knowledge and expertise required for comprehensive general medical care to expect such knowledge and expertise to exist in small groups. Exceptions apply to very focused areas of medicine, such as dermatology and dentistry, where small groups (even individuals) may be effective.

Groups of providers that are too large (> 160 members) will continually fail to provide quality, cost-efficient care because of the time and energy devoted to within-group competition and communication (e.g., excessive meetings) and the difficulties encountered in monitoring and influencing the behavior of group members. Hierarchies, inelastic interaction systems, and constraints on free information flow not only characterize large groups, but they also cost too much money. As the number of persons in a group increases, so does the number of rules and the importance placed on following them, regardless of their value to those persons the system is supposed to serve. In such an environment, quality of care, provider morale, agreed upon shared rules, internal monitoring, and specificity of purpose decline while uncertainty increases. Furthermore, the distance between decision makers and patients increases as decisions about medical care are progressively taken out of the hands of providers and left to administrators and their preoccupations with costs, profits, statistical data, the management of large numbers of individuals, and their own status. Such activities divert energy and interest away from patient care. They are costly. They compromise purpose.

Groups of medium size (26–160 individuals) are groups in which: (1) individuals can make special contributions; (2) there can be valuable divisions of labor based on skills and knowledge; (3) there can be enough expert knowledge to address optimally the vast majority of medical problems; (4) there can be a high degree of internal review and monitoring; (5) communication can be efficient; (6) others' behavior is well known and can be influenced; (7) there can be a high degree of social responsibility; (8) pay can be based on merit; (9) members can take responsibility for resource use and distribution; (10) members can take responsibility for medical errors; and (11) costs can be contained. Most important, opportunities for within-group reciprocal relationships are optimized.

Groups of medium size are consistent with the basic proclivities of human nature. Humans have evolved as members of medium size groups and it is in such groups that they function optimally. Nowhere is this point more clear than in communication. Much of critical within-group information can be transmitted efficiently by word of mouth and remembered. Manuals and memos take on secondary importance.

## SCENARIOS

How might the points above unfold in different healthcare systems? Seven scenarios are considered. Scenario 1 deals with a small healthcare group, Scenario 2 with a large healthcare group, Scenario 3 with an HMO, Scenario 4 with a health insurance company, Scenario 5 with a government healthcare facility, Scenario 6 with a medium-size local healthcare group, and Scenario 7 with a medium-size community-based healthcare group.

### Scenario 1—A Small Healthcare Group

Twenty healthcare personnel work in a private healthcare facility and attempt to treat patients except for those requiring highly specialized treatment (e.g., lung transplants). Payments for services are contracted through insurance companies, Medicare, direct and co-payment, and Medicaid.

*Potential positive features of Scenario 1 include*: (1) The accurate identification of most diseases and disorders. (2) Adequate treatment of most diseases. (3) Providers as important members of the system. (4) Focus of purpose. (5) Optimization of communication. (6) Minimization of administrative meetings. (7) Containment of costs is possible. (8) Cooperation between the patients and providers can occur. (9) Within-group monitoring of quality of care can occur. (10) Within-group decisions about healthcare resource allocation can occur. (11) Continuity of care can occur. (12) Sensitivity to individual differences can occur.

*Potential negative features of Scenario 1 include*: (1) A percentage of diseases will not be recognized because of the lack of required expertise. (2) Limitations on the variety of diseases that can be treated. (3) Function less than optimal because of lack of expertise. (4) Function also limited, and often significantly, by decisions made by third-party payers (e.g., insurance companies may discontinue contracts, Medicare may set criteria for treatment, etc). (5) No assurance that patients will influence cost of care, cost containment, or quality of healthcare delivery. (6) No assurance that patients' expectations will be met. (7) Provider income flow moderately uncertain. (8) Patient willingness to pay for medical care will vary in response to the quality and availability of care.

### Scenario 2—A Large Healthcare Group

Six hundred healthcare personnel work in a large community hospital and treat patients with all types of diseases. Payments for their services are contracted through insurance companies, direct and co-payment, Medicare, and Medicaid.

*Potential positive features of Scenario 2 include*: (1) The percentage of diseases that will not be recognized because of the lack of expertise will be less than with Scenario 1. (2) Limitations on the number of treatable diseases less than with Scenario 1. (3) Provider income flow improved over Scenario 1.

*Potential negative features of Scenario 2 include*: (1) Cooperation between players will be time consuming and difficult because of the unfamiliarity of many players, competition for resources, and differing agendas. (2) Focus of purpose compromised because of diverse interest of providers. (3) Communication inefficient and frequent reinforcement required (e.g., frequent within-discipline and cross-discipline administrative meetings). (4) Quality of care reduced compared to Scenario 1. (5) Containment of costs difficult because of the different requirements in different specialties. (6) Within-group monitoring of quality of care cumbersome and inefficient because of the large number of members in the group and because the details of different specialties are not well known to many group members. (7) Within-group decisions about healthcare resource allocation often adversarial and influenced by power structure. (8) Continuity of care seldom fully achieved. (9) Function limited, often significantly, by within-group and cross-group competition as well as by decisions made by third-party payers. (10) Minimal patient influence on cost of care, quality of healthcare delivery, and choice of individual providers. (11) Less assurance than in Scenario 1 that patients' predispositions will be met. (12) Patient willingness to pay for medical care less than in Scenario 1. (13) Increased chance of insensitivity to individual differences and expectations.

### Scenario 3—An HMO

Thirty-five hundred healthcare personnel are employed by an HMO with six hospitals and associated outpatient clinics. Payments to the HMO are received through clients and in some instances through Medicare contracts.

*Many of the potential positive and negative features of Scenario 3* are similar to those of Scenario 2. There are important exceptions, however. (1) In many HMOs, there is less continuity of care. (2) Quality of care is likely to be reduced compared to Scenario 2 (e.g., patients treated as statistical entities rather than individuals).[10] (3) Patients have minimal influence on quality of care and care delivery. (4) Providers have less control over medical decisions and income. (5) Internal monitoring is largely outside of the hands of providers. (6) Containment of costs outside of the hands of providers and patients, and costs per service increased because of the need to support the administrative structure of large businesses and the need for profits. (7) Focus of purpose determined by administrators. (8) Cooperation among administrators and providers compromised. (9) Communication more authoritarian and inflexible. (10) Decisions about healthcare resource allocation outside of the hands of providers and patients. (11) Greater compromises in quality of care. (12) Patient willingness to pay increased fees for medical care less than in either Scenario 1 or 2.

### Scenario 4—A Health Insurance Company

Six thousand healthcare personnel are preferred providers to an insurance company with all types of diseases covered. Providers receive payments for their services through the insurance company which collects payments from members of their healthcare system.

*Potential positive features of Scenario 4 include*: (1) For a small percentage of persons, catastrophic medical costs are covered by insurance. (2) Continuity of care is a possibility.

*Potential negative features of Scenario 4 include*: (1) Need for profit constrains provider–patient options. (2) Cooperation between patients, providers, and insurers time consuming, difficult, and often adversarial. (3) Communication among providers inefficient and communication duplication required because players are not well known to each other. (4) Quality of care variable and differs significantly across providers and insurance companies but usually less than Scenarios 1 and 2. (5) Important healthcare decisions may be made by individuals who are not medically knowledgeable. (6) Cost containment and resource allocation determined almost entirely by insurance company personnel (e.g., cross-specialty referrals usually constrained). (7) Monitoring of provider quality difficult because of the number of providers and the number of different specialties. (8) Quality of care less than optimal because of conflicts among players and cost containment. (9) Minimal patient influence on cost of care, cost containment, quality of healthcare delivery, and choice of individual providers. (10) Patient and provider predispositions relatively inconsequential. (11) Patient willingness to pay for medical care less than in Scenarios 1 and 2.

### Scenario 5—A Government Health Facility

The Veterans Administration medical service can be used as a model of a government healthcare facility. The Veterans Administration employs literally thousands of healthcare personnel in a bureaucratic and highly hierarchical organization which, over the last two decades, has been in a state of continual change.[11]

Some historical points will be valuable here. Prior to World War II, Veterans Administration healthcare had established itself as a high-quality although expensive healthcare system which devoted itself to the veterans from World War I and those enlisted personnel who were injured or who became sick between World War I and World War II. With World War II, the need for far more expanded medical and rehabilitation services was undisputed by both the government and the citizens of the United States. Following World War II, the veterans' healthcare system expanded significantly. For the subsequent three and a half decades, wars in Korea and Viet Nam added to the need for healthcare services. However, the need for such services began to decline in the late 1980s. Fewer World War II veterans were alive. Those injured in Korea and Viet Nam were either treated or had moved to a chronic patient status. And Operation Desert Storm resulted in relatively few new casualities.

Also in the 1980s, the first signs of size reduction in the Veterans Administration began to surface. Healthcare facilities located throughout the country were expensive to maintain and Congress wanted to use the monies elsewhere. The trimming of the Veterans Administration budget began. As it did, the top echelons of the system remained in place, but from the late 1980s to the early 1990s there was a disproportionate decline in the number of providers and their support services. The administrative structure of the Veterans Administration remained intact. Only in the mid-1990s did the administrative structure begin seriously to trim its staff and to accommodate for the declining funds.

There is a lesson to be learned from this history: Once a bureaucratic system is in place, the administrative arm of the bureaucracy is likely to attempt to preserve itself despite the consequences to those it supposedly serves. Similar scenarios can be imagined for insurance companies, HMOs, and the government over the next two decades.

*Potential positive features of Scenario 5 include:* (1) The percentage of diseases that will be unrecognized because of the lack of expertise will be less than with Scenario 1. (2) In principle, limitations on the variety of diseases treated will be less than with Scenario 1. Practice, however, may be another matter. (3) In principle, cross-specialty referrals are facilitated, although at this point it often takes several months for a referral to be honored. (4) Healthcare costs to veterans are usually nonexistent or low, especially to veterans injured in action.

*Potential negative features of Scenario 5 include*: (1) Cooperation between the players is difficult, especially at the clinical level. This is due largely to the competition for resources among providers as well as among remotely located Veterans Administration hospitals. (2) Cooperation between the patients and providers is time consuming and difficult to achieve, primarily because providers change frequently. (3) Focus of purpose is difficult because of the diverse interest of the Veterans Administration and providers, the fact that the Veterans Administration must account to Congress, and the fact that there are a variety of interest groups (e.g., VFW) representing veterans. (4) Communication is inefficient and communication backups are required because players are not well known to each other. (5) Quality of care is reduced compared to Scenario 1 due to frequent changes in the Veterans Administration hierarchical structure, the goals of clinical care, and changes in providers. (6) Within-discipline and cross-discipline administrative meetings are frequent, due to the need to deal with the often changing and complex decision-making structure of the Veterans Administration. (7) Containment of costs is enforced from above but not necessarily efficient or relevant (e.g., decisions are often made by persons not familiar with the details of medical care). (8) Within-group monitoring of quality of care is difficult because of the number of members in the group, because the details of different specialties are not well known to all group members, and because regulations make within-group monitoring costly in terms of time and within-group consequences. (9) Within-group decisions about resource allocation are cumbersome and often adversarial. (10) Continuity of care is significantly limited because of provider turnover. (11) Quality of care is significantly less than optimal because of time devoted to administration, communication, responding to requirements imposed from "above" (Central Office of the Veterans Administration), and resource—related competition. (12) Minimal patient influence on quality of care, cost of care, cost containment, delivery of care, and choice of individual providers. (13) Minimal patient influence over the degree to which their predispositions are met.

## Scenario 6—A Medium-Sized Healthcare Group

One hundred and thirty-five healthcare personnel work in a community healthcare facility and treat patients with all types of medical illnesses. Payments for their services are contracted through insurance companies, direct payment, Medicare, and Medicaid.

*Potential positive features of Scenario 6* are similar to Scenario 1, but there are distinct advantages over Scenario 1. (1) Accurate identification of most diseases greater than Scenario 1. (2) Capacity to treat most diseases greater than Scenario 1. (3) Greater cooperation between patients and providers likely. (4) Providers more likely to be important members of the system. (5) Focus of purpose likely. (6) Optimization of communication among players.

(7) Minimization of administrative meetings. (8) Containment of costs. (9) Within-group monitoring of quality. (10) Within-group decisions about healthcare resource allocation a possibility. (11) Continuity of care likely. (12) Cross-discipline referrals facilitated. (13) Close to optimal functioning a possibility.

*Potential negative features of Scenario 6 include:* (1) A relatively small percentage of diseases (less than Scenario 1) will go unrecognized, and the degree of recognition will depend on two factors: the number of hands-on providers and the number of providers who review complex cases. (2) Relatively few limitations on the variety of diseases that can be treated. Those that cannot be treated will usually require the assistance of larger facilities such as university hospitals that often have large numbers of experts in specific areas, advanced technology, and the technology to treat difficult medical problems (e.g., radiation therapy, complex surgical procedures). (3) Decisions made by third-party payers may compromise the quality of care. (4) Provider income flow may fluctuate. (5) Patient willingness to pay for medical care will depend on the degree to which patients can influence the operation of the system.

### Scenario 7—A Community-Based Healthcare Group in which Patients and Providers Are the Key Decision Makers

This is a variation of Scenario 6 in which both patients and providers actively participate in the decision making and administration of the system and there is a variety of payment possibilities. Two features distinguish this type of group from Scenario 6: novel modes of payment and the degree of patient and provider participation.

Community members would be able to pay for their care by several methods including: (1) government payments (applicable primarily to the elderly); (2) buying health insurance from the facility (which would reinsure itself); (3) directly (through medical savings accounts); or (4) service to the healthcare group. Patient and provider participation would focus on decisions dealing with quality of care, resource allocation, treatment priorities, and the type of care offered. In effect, individuals in a community would determine the type of healthcare they want, how they would pay for it, and how they would administer it.

A comment about healthcare insurance and reinsurance. We have argued strongly that insurance companies which insure individuals for their day-to-day healthcare costs are a major impediment to quality healthcare. Administrative-management costs are high. Database disease management is common. Patients and providers are often required to assume adversarial positions with respect to healthcare claims. The same points need not apply to reinsurance. For example, a community-based healthcare group could insure itself against medical costs for costs that exceed a specified amount.

Reinsurance would protect the community-based group from financial collapse.[12,13]

*Potential positive features of Scenario 7* are similar to Scenario 6 but offer additional healthcare advantages. (1) The accurate identification of most diseases is equivalent to Scenario 6. (2) Treatment of most diseases is equivalent to Scenario 6. (3) Cooperation between the patients and providers can exceed Scenario 6. (4) Providers feeling that they are important members of the healthcare system is more likely than in Scenario 6. (5) Focus of purpose more likely than Scenario 6. (6) Optimization of communication among all players a definite possibility. (7) Minimization of administrative meetings. (8) Containment of costs a definite possibility. (9) Within-group monitoring of quality of care a real possibility because players are known to each other. (10) Within-group decisions about healthcare resource allocation a real possibility. (11) Continuity of care a definite possibility. (12) Cross-unit referrals facilitated. (13) Greatest chance for optimal functioning compared to any of the other scenarios. (14) Quality of care minimally compromised by third-party insurance or federal and state government, and HMO-type problems avoided. (15) Patient willingness to pay for care is higher than in any of the other scenarios. (16) The chances of predisposition being optimized the greatest of any of the scenarios.

*Potential negative features of Scenario 7 include*: (1) A relatively small percentage of diseases will not be recognized, as in Scenario 6. (2) Relatively few limitations on the variety of diseases that can be treated, as Scenario 6—and those that cannot be treated can be sent to other facilities.

Increased patient and provider participation in healthcare decisions deserves some additional explanation. A reasonable expectation is that there will continue to be limits to the amount of resources available for healthcare. Given such limits, a key question becomes: "Who will decide how the resources are allocated?" While all resource allocation plans have limitations, it is our view that the most realistic and satisfactory solution to the allocation issue is to place it in the hands of persons in the community rather than turn it over to federal or state governments or let the marketplace decide.

## LIKELY RESPONSES TO THESE RECOMMENDATIONS

What are the likely reactions among various parties to our recommendations, particularly to the idea that the most optimal healthcare system is a medium-size system, not a large system, not a small system?

- The majority of patients will respond favorably because of the opportunity to participate in decisions about their own care as well as the care of kin and community members. This will have the effect of reducing uncertainty, optimizing continuity of care and ease of access to healthcare providers, and increasing reciprocity.

- The majority of hands-on healthcare providers will respond favorably because of their participation in the decision-making aspects of care delivery, because of the reduction in activities that take away from hands-on care, and the satisfaction that accrues from continuity of care.

- Medical administrators and entrepreneurs will oppose the recommendations because their jobs and profits would be in jeopardy.

- Lawyers will oppose our recommendations because as cooperation increases the probability of lawsuits against providers decreases.

- HMOs would be unhappy because they will be phased out of business.

- The government dominated by Democrats will be skeptical and oppose our recommendations. A government dominated by Republicans will be supportive.

## NOTES

1. See an article by B. Coleman in the *Fresno Bee*, 28 July 1997, for a summary of workplace injury statistics in America during the last year: 6,500 deaths and 13,200,000 work-related injuries.

2. See an article by J. Calmes in the *Wall Street Journal*, 10 February 1997. The author summarizes the current population projections for the elderly: persons of age 66 and older are predicted to rise from, 18,000,000+ in the year 2000 to 37,000,000+ in 2030.

3. M. Langley, in the *Wall Street Journal*, 2 May 1997, reports on how at some locations Columbia/HCA is requiring doctors to end their outside practices.

4. One of our postulates has been that a root cause of healthcare difficulty is our overreliance on insurance. R. Brownstein, *Los Angeles Times*, 7 April 1997, reports on how, with increasing confidence, conservative thinkers are challenging the principle that collective insurance offers the most secure retirement to Americans.

5. See R. Brownstein, "Prescription for Medicare Reform Could Have Unexpected Side Effects," *Los Angeles Times*, 7 July 1997. The author documents some of the likely side effects of planned changes in Medicare, including higher fees to the elderly.

6. San Francisco is considering universal healthcare coverage. See S. Heinoff, "Falling to Safety," *California Medicine*, July 1997.

7. Diagnostic precision is frequently elusive, even in common and serious illnesses. See, for example, M. Cimons, "Breast Cancer Study Offers Hope but No Easy Answers," *Los Angeles Times*, 7 April 1998. The author addresses the complexity and elusiveness of diagnosing and treating breast cancer.

8. One resource often overlooked is the place of charitable foundations in the healthcare mosaic. See K. Mills, "On the Role of Health Foundations in Caring for California's Poor," *Los Angeles Times*, 29 March 1998.

9. There is a tendency in human decision making to assume that information that is difficult to acquire is probably not that important. See J. E. Rein, "Misinformation and Self-Deception in Recent Long-Term Care Policy Trends," *Journal of Law and Politics* 12 (1996): 195–340. Self-deception contributes to the chaos of health policy.

10. Current HMO strategy attempts to replace people of extensive education and

training with others of lesser educational experience. See an article by R. Winslow in the *Wall Street Journal*, 7 February 1997. The author documents how Oxford Health Plans, Inc., plans to turn over to nurses many duties traditionally handled by doctors at the Columbia Presbyterian Medical Center.

11. See W. Poole, "The VA's Last Stand," *California Medicine*, June 1997, in which the author documents how the Veterans Administration healthcare system is changing in response to market-driven forms.

12. See C. Georges, *Wall Street Journal*, 15 May 1997, for an analysis of the positive effects of the Iowa welfare system, in which most people who go off the system manage to succeed.

13. One example of community involvement from the world of sports may be instructive. R. Wilson, in an unpublished manuscript entitled "Community Benefits Forestry," cites the wonderful financial and other types of success of the Green Bay Packers and how this success is tied to offering stock to the local community.

# Chapter 12

# Fifty-One
# Questions and Answers

**QUESTION 1:**

Is there a root cause for our discontent about the current system of healthcare?

**ANSWER:**

In our view a great deal of the problem can be traced to our tendency to insist that insurance be the main means by which costs are covered. This form of prepayment is appropriate for major and unexpected illness and injury, but when used for routine matters it causes us to be insensitive to costs and indifferent to potential savings. This prepayment scheme at first encourages overutilization, and later promotes efforts to control escalating costs by various measures to ration service. Prepaid healthcare thus promotes increased costs and reduced access and quality. As noted in an earlier chapter, in order to see how prepaid healthcare works, it is a useful exercise to imagine what would happen to our diets if we had a system of prepaid grocery service. At first we would buy too much caviar and champagne, and later the store would have to restrict us to cheap, nutritious gruel.

**QUESTION 2:**

But what alternative is there to prepaid care through insurance?

**ANSWER:**

Unexpected and catastrophic expenses should be covered by insurance. Elective and routine care should be covered by out-of-pocket payment, just as other necessities are, such as food, clothing, housing, and car maintenance. One way to make this easier would be to fold in a medical savings account with the catastrophic insurance. Such accounts could be authorized by government mandate and would receive regular monthly payments by payroll deduction. These funds could be invested in a conservative growth portfolio that would, with compounding of interest, grow to be able to fund much of the care we need as we grow older. Costs would be controlled by the market discipline that occurs when we pay for something with money that we see as our own. We as individuals would regain control of the process of healthcare. Providers would begin to work for us again.

## QUESTION 3:

Every other advanced country has some form of government health service which guarantees healthcare to everyone. Why shouldn't we go in that direction?

## ANSWER:

This health plan, in whatever scheme is devised, makes the government into a big insurance company. The same problems arise, but it takes longer to discover them because the government has deep pockets. First, there is overuse of services and later there is rationing. When we have the illusion that a service is free, this is the inevitable sequence of events. Worse, the government has a monopoly on force, and so it may at last dictate what care is available and who gets it. In the final analysis, the government owns our bodies. True, other advanced countries have gone down this road, and most of their citizens have approved the services they have received. But as healthcare has become more complex these governmental plans have begun to unravel, with various forms of care restriction becoming necessary. We believe it is better for free people to make their own decisions on these intimate matters.

## QUESTION 4:

Shouldn't healthcare be considered a right?

## ANSWER:

We don't think so. We believe this is a political slogan rather than a well-reasoned position. We think this slogan clouds our thinking about solutions in the real world. Healthcare is not a commodity. You simply cannot give an equal number of scoops of it to everyone. Some people want a lot, and others a little. Some people need a lot, and others a little. These are not always the same people. To imagine healthcare as a right is to ensure that rationing, quality decrease, and access limitation will eventually occur. To insist that care be uniformly distributed is to guarantee that other mechanisms of exchange will occur, such as bribery, barter, or political corruption.

## QUESTION 5:

But shouldn't everyone be treated equally?

## ANSWER:

Everyone should be. The operative question is how best to do that. Everyone should have equal access to the same standard of quality care. At the same time, we believe it is essential that patients exercise effective control over the diagnostic and therapeutic process, and take responsibility for these decisions. Patients, whenever possible, should pay for their care with money that they see as theirs. For patients who do not have adequate resources to accomplish this, government assistance is appropriate. As noted, this assistance could be given in a form where a patient's control of the process would be retained. For example, an account analogous to a medical savings account could be provided with a fixed sum available on a yearly basis; the disbursement would be at the patient's discretion. Such an account, together with catastrophic insurance, would promote individual autonomy and responsibility. Delivery systems organized around communities could also provide care on a charitable basis.

## QUESTION 6:

But do all patients have sufficient judgment to exercise this autonomy? Might they not waste their account money on frivolous or ineffective treatments?

## ANSWER:

They might, but it is their money to waste. Any system of payment runs this risk. It is not at all clear that having someone else (even the government) make these decisions for you necessarily leads to wiser choices. We believe that, over time, good practice will prevail. For those who are truly mentally compromised, the current system of guardianship or medical power of attorney seems appropriate.

## QUESTION 7:

But still, won't care tend to be unequally distributed?

**ANSWER:**

It will. Nothing can change that, since care is always driven by the particular illness or disease in question. Some people are luckier and healthier than others. The important concept is equally available access to care.

## QUESTION 8:

Shouldn't the government control healthcare costs?

**ANSWER:**

No. All attempts at price control are ultimately unstable and produce shortages of valuable goods and services as well as surpluses of those less valued. There is no reason to believe that healthcare might be different in this regard. As in every other area of economic life, the truly free market gives a better resource allocation than any ad hoc scheme people are likely to devise. The task is to devise a system in which the market can be as free as possible. As in so many other areas of human activity, perfection continues to elude us, but some methods are superior to others.

## QUESTION 9:

Whom do you consider the interested parties in the solution of the problems of healthcare?

**ANSWER:**

Healthcare is fundamentally a contractual relationship between patients and professional providers. Patients' families also have an important interest. Insurance companies and government have an ancillary enabling role by providing a financial environment which fosters a maximum of patient responsibility and autonomy.

## QUESTION 10:

What is the real cause of the escalation of healthcare costs far beyond the rate of inflation?

**ANSWER:**

In general, costs are controlled by the free market, with a myriad of individual decisions bringing supply and demand into equilibrium. When paying for goods or services is separated by space and time from receiving them, then the free market becomes inefficient at best. One simple example is the tendency for people to spend more than they can afford when they have access to a major credit card. Another is the explosion of costs of higher education as federally guaranteed loans have become available. But the clearest example is in healthcare, where insurance availability has created the illusion that care is free or has been prepaid in full, regardless of the expense or demand. When a valuable commodity or service is perceived as free, prices tend to escalate.

## QUESTION 11:

But doesn't the explosion of technological advances drive costs up? Wouldn't it be appropriate for government to put curbs on the expansion of technology?

## ANSWER:

Curbing technology would be the height of folly. In literally every other area of human experience, advancement of science and technology has brought about both an increase in the total wealth of a society and a broader distribution of the wealth. Technology makes goods cheaper, more available, and higher in quality. Why should medical care delivery be different? True, in the case of medical care, technology has not made services cheaper, although they are more available and higher in quality. This is explained by the set of distorted incentives brought on by a failure in market discipline. In a price-sensitive environment, advances in technology would have the effect of improving quality, availability, and cost.

## QUESTION 12:

But improvements in technology mean that the number of diagnostic and treatment options increase. Won't this have the inevitable effect of increasing total medical costs?

## ANSWER:

It will. And this is a good thing. The goal of healthcare is not to avoid all cost increases, but rather to avoid those not accompanied by proportional increase in productivity and quality. Once the average American worker earned less than a dollar an hour. The increases in labor costs we have experienced in this century have been accompanied by even larger increases in productivity, and wealth for all has proportionally been enhanced. Antibiotics increased the costs of healthcare, but few would wish to go back to the cheap "good old days" before we had them. The question is not merely whether costs increase, but whether we are getting our money's worth. If we place limits on future growth of technology, then why not ban the advances we have recently gained? And where do we start? Renal dialysis? Ask someone with kidney failure. Heart surgery? Ask someone with severe angina.

## QUESTION 13:

But isn't insurance coverage the only way that today's costs can be affordable?

## ANSWER:

Insurance increases costs. Still, it useful and desirable for coverage of those costs which are unexpected, unusual, or catastrophic. But to use insurance to pay for routine matters is to guarantee cost increases in excess of productivity.

## QUESTION 14:

Why have "alternative" means of treatment recently begun to enjoy such an enormous increase in popularity?

## ANSWER:

Alternative treatments have existed in uneasy association with scientific medicine for a very long time. The forms are myriad. Homeopathy, herbalism, acupuncture, chiropractic, therapeutic touch, and psychic healing are some of the more popular current offerings. Some of them, sometimes, may have some actual benefits. What distinguishes them from mainstream or scientific medicine is the absence of controlled clinical trials which might be able to demonstrate efficacy in replicable ways. Some of these alternatives are not testable. Others are testable in principle, but when trials are attempted, they fail to show therapeutic value. Failure to attract scientific support does not deter their advocates and practitioners from continued avid use of them. Still, they have one important advantage over mainstream treatments—they are readily available and not, in general, subject to restriction and denial by managed care organizations and other providers. Many of us seem to be willing to engage in faith or wishful thinking in order to have what seems to be control over the way we are treated.

## QUESTION 15:

A large fraction of our lifetime medical care costs occurs in the last year of our lives. Is this a proper use of resources?

## ANSWER:

This is a question full of logical and moral quicksand. First of all, as owners of own bodies, it is in the last analysis up to each of us individually to decide how to allocate these resources. But that aside, how can we know in advance whether we have entered that last expensive year? Of course a lot of costs accrue in the last year. That is usually when we are sickest! What is the alternative? Shall we put our sick older citizens on an ice floe and push them out to sea? Patients have a right to decide these most intimate matters.

## QUESTION 16:

How important is confidentiality in medical treatment?

## ANSWER:

Some people view absolute confidentiality as supremely important. Others view it as one of several criteria of good care. Still others see it as only secondary in importance. But whatever one's opinion, it is by now clear that insurance coverage generally, and managed care plans in particular, have entirely vitiated the practice of confidentiality. Seldom are patients aware of the amount or sensitivity of the information a medical record may contain, or the number of people who may gain access to it with anonymity and impunity. Not only are diagnoses to be reported to third-party payers, but so are all the data necessary to support the diagnoses and the recommended treatments. Physicians may be interrogated by clerks with no hesitation to ask the most penetrating questions. If the physician demurs, the third party may threaten to decline payment. Patients are thus easily coerced into signing comprehensive waivers of confidentiality. The conclusion is unavoidable: confidentiality may exist only to the extent that patients pay for their care directly.

## QUESTION 17:

How can I afford to pay for healthcare by myself?

## ANSWER:

Most of us pay for it ourselves now, and then some. In doing so, we support a large superstructure of factotums, functionaries, regulators, assessors, clerks, lawyers, advertising personnel, chief executive officers, and stockholders. Their services often add up to 30%–40% of the costs, and this may be an underestimate; much of their work introduces indirect costs related to interaction with one another. One of the results of this superstructure is to create the illusion that care is not affordable without their help. We can afford our own healthcare using a combination of catastrophic insurance, medical savings accounts, community organizations, barter, local charity, and government grants-in-aid to the medically indigent.

## QUESTION 18:

How can fraud, waste, and abuse be minimized?

## ANSWER:

Although cheating and free riding are, unfortunately, part of the human experience, there are some organizational ways in which they can be minimized. In general, people tend toward the greatest degree of honesty and fair dealing when they work with their own kin. Blood is, as has been said, thicker than water. But most of the time this condition does not prevail during transactions surrounding healthcare. The next best situation is to work in groups which, although not related, nevertheless have formed emotional and reciprocal ties among themselves. Still, this is not always practical in the medical environment. What we can do is arrange groups of affiliated providers known to each other personally, thus having some shared and mutually perceived responsibility to act honorably. These groups of providers should not exceed a certain size. Groups of about 100 are sufficiently small; all participants should know each other personally so as to form affiliative bonds. Close relationships reduce the likelihood of cheating.

## QUESTION 19:

What is the Hippocratic Oath?

## ANSWER:

The Hippocratic Oath is a solemn promise made by physicians for the past 2,400 years to conduct their personal and professional lives with uprightness and honor, requiring members to work solely for the benefit of the patient, to avoid any doing of harm, and in particular, never to prescribe a deadly drug, to avoid seduction of patients, and to preserve confidentiality. Serving as the cornerstone of medical ethics in the Western tradition from ancient times, it does not require physicians to accept any patient who requests care, nor does it say that patients should not be required to pay. Although not always perfectly observed, the Hippocratic Oath remains an honored ideal to which physicians properly aspire. In the last half century, it has come under attack as being insensitive to social consciousness—that is, by centering its concerns on the individual patient, it implicitly denies that the good of society should be of greater importance. The twentieth century has been one long experiment in the applications of variations on this theme. The currently popular incarnation of this idea is that the managed care organization, as the representative of society, should come first in the physician's hierarchy of concerns.

## QUESTION 20:

What about malpractice?

## ANSWER:

Two related problems must be considered separately in a discussion of malpractice. One is the legitimate concern about negligence or substandard practice on the part of professionals; these problems must be identified and corrected. The other is that occasionally an unfortunate result occurs in spite of careful and appropriate treatment. A difficulty arises when the two are confused. Compensation to the patient for injury occurring in spite of good treatment should be made by insurance specific to that purpose. Compensation resulting from actual negligence or substandard care should be borne at the expense of the offending professional, probably through the mediation of professional liability insurance. The real problem is to identify which is which. If substandard practice is effectively mandated by a third party such as an HMO, then the organization should bear the costs. One advantage of payment by means of medical savings accounts is that the physician has greater incentive to explain treatment decisions in detail and thus share the responsibility with the patient. The result is likely to be fewer frivolous lawsuits.

## QUESTION 21:

How much money should professionals make?

## ANSWER:

Professionals should earn what a truly free market would determine when supply and demand are in balance. The problem is one of promoting a system which allows for this ideal free market to flourish. In general, people who have more talent, more education and training, more responsibility, and longer hours expect to be paid more. But it is possible that many tasks do not require the attention of a supremely trained specialist. The only way that we know of for a stable system of compensation to evolve is for people to get what they pay for, and be well informed about what services they truly need or want. Neither government nor professional organizations should put artificial constraint on the number of practitioners. The purpose of these external regulators should be to specify standards of quality, not quantity.

## QUESTION 22:

What is the role of teaching hospitals?

## ANSWER:

Certain hospitals need to be staffed and equipped to treat the most unusual and complicated cases. We need to train medical students and medical specialists. It makes good sense to do both these tasks in the same places, the tertiary care centers, or "teaching hospitals." Costs are, of course, higher in these places, for the simple reason that complicated cases require more intensive care, and teaching is not an optimally efficient activity. One problem as yet unsolved is the best means to cover the extra costs of this education and intensive treatment. Currently, in many places, hospitals with resident training programs receive a per capita subsidy for each trainee. This practice has the unfortunate consequence of creating the perverse incentive to create training programs where none are needed, or to enlarge existing programs beyond the expected needs for specialists. As is always the case, subsidies create surpluses. This, in turn, means we could have more specialists than we need, and training may not be always of the highest quality. We have to find a better way than this. Of course, teaching hospitals should command a premium fee structure when (and if) the cases they treat are indeed more complicated; part of this premium might pay the training costs.

## QUESTION 23:

What about continuing education for professionals?

## ANSWER:

Rapid scientific advances in medicine require all professionals to receive regular and intensive updating of their knowledge and skills. It seems reasonable for the professionals themselves to bear the expense of this activity. In most cases, it is probably appropriate to utilize medical and nursing schools as loci of these activities. It is important that no special arrangements be made for financial subsidy, lest perverse incentives again appear, and educational activities of dubious quality and excess quantity appear. By the same token, enough sites should be available for competition to exist in a meaningful way in order to keeps costs in balance with value received.

QUESTION 24:

How do your proposals differ from previous ideas?

ANSWER:

We attempt to build on what we see as the best emerging ideas, such as medical savings accounts. We think the missing ingredient has been the failure to consider the essence of human nature, and its tendency to cause cooperation, competition, or contentiousness. Depending on critical variables such as the size of the group in question and the degree of emotional attachment and affiliation within it, people behave in predictable ways. Humans respond to incentives, and we work hard to circumvent rules. Thus, it seems to us, the unit of healthcare organization ought to be small enough to have members feel some mutual responsibility and enjoy effective communication on a personal basis. This, we think, would cause the system to evolve toward greater quality and efficiency, while reducing cheating and thus reducing costs.

QUESTION 25:

What would organizing healthcare in this way require?

ANSWER:

The first step is the permission of federal and state governments to begin experimental trials of organizations of providers. Tax exempt medical savings accounts would have to be authorized on a large-scale basis. Insurance companies would have to be encouraged to offer combinations of catastrophic insurance compatible with these slowly growing accounts. Patients would have to be recruited by demonstrating to them how a new mode of delivery would be superior to the procrustean healthcare system currently offered in the managed care environment.

QUESTION 26:

What time frame might be required?

ANSWER:

We do not see our proposals as time critical. If we are right, that there is a better way to organize care, one that is a more natural fit with the human propensity to follow incentives and to cooperate effectively when in groups of the right size, then small pilot experiments would quickly duplicate themselves at the grass-roots level. We think such groups could compete with currently available delivery systems. Group systems for healthcare will spread quickly to the extent that their superiority is clear.

## QUESTION 27:

How would your pilot programs handle the problem of free riders, such as those pretending to be indigents or transients?

## ANSWER:

We don't think this will be a large-scale problem during the early pilot trials. Emergencies involving transients or uninsured nonmembers can be managed as a necessary service in the Hippocratic tradition. If and when the provider groups become a significant fraction of the national delivery system, there will be a need to make provisions for the contingency of free riders. Our point is not that the plan we advance is perfect, but only that it is better prepared to deal with problems of this type, since its underlying principles are more consistent with what is known of the behavior of people in groups.

## QUESTION 28:

How would quality of professional practitioners and institutions be monitored and assessed?

## ANSWER:

We think the mechanisms currently in place are adequate in principle, but they could be more effective in a framework where all the practitioners in a group are responsible to each other on a personal basis for the quality of the service that they provide. Peer review would be the main way that quality is monitored. When groups are large, quality measurements take on a formalistic style, strong on procedure and often short on meaningful content. When no one knows anyone else, peer review would be reduced to examination of the completeness of records. While this is, of course, important, it contains the regrettable incentive to spend more time on enhancing the appearance of the record than on the delivery of high-quality care. Federal and state licensing authorities would continue their scrutiny, as would a drastically revised JCAHO—one that is designed to deal with medically relevant issues rather than fads or its own perpetuation.

## QUESTION 29:

How would the delivery system you describe be likely to have an impact on some of the current ethical debates, such as the purported right to physician-assisted suicide?

## ANSWER:

We believe the effect would be salubrious. Ethical decisions exist within the interstices of the law, typically residing in ambiguous areas in which facts and values interact in a murky way. It is not easy to define methods of approach to these difficult but supremely important problems. On balance, it seems to us, that these problems are best examined by those closest to the facts. This suggests that a small organization may be superior to a large one for this purpose.

## QUESTION 30:

What about the working poor?

## ANSWER:

People with low incomes may have, at any given time, less money in their medical savings accounts than people with high incomes. This problem is similar to that of the equal distribution of other necessities, such as food and shelter. It could be managed the same way. For example, tax credits could be given to those whose income is below a certain amount, thus allowing for enhanced contributions to the account.

## QUESTION 31:

Still, will this not mean that some low-income people will have less discretionary money in their medical savings accounts?

## ANSWER:

Yes it will, just as they may have less money for food and housing. If we thought it possible to design a system of utopian equality, we would gladly have done so. But history suggests that such attempts invariably have seriously flawed and unintended consequences. Too often, the twentieth century has suffered from various experiments in that regard. We recognize that the course we suggest is not perfect; nevertheless, our plan would be a large improvement over the current situation. Final achievement of perfect equality will require divine intervention, which does not now appear in sight.

## QUESTION 32:

Sometimes it seems as though we are becoming a nation of victims. How will this social phenomenon influence the course of healthcare?

## ANSWER:

The modern affluent American society appears to have created a "niche" in which some of us attempt to enhance our position or status by claiming special rights on the basis of an imputed or imagined prior unfair treatment. To pursue this strategy it must follow that personal responsibility must be denied or abandoned. The inevitable end of this course is to abdicate duty to self, family, and community and become, in effect, a domestic animal, dependent on the state for whatever benefits there might be. A free society cannot survive in the long run if the number of ostensible victims exceeds some critical threshold. Thus we expect that taking more responsibility for our own healthcare decisions and organizing care around the community is not only the most efficient way, but it is also the most patriotic way.

## QUESTION 33:

How does the local community fit into your plan?

## ANSWER:

We think the community is most likely to be the right size to maximize efficiencies for the same reasons that groups of providers need to be the right size. When people have formed emotional attachments, they are less likely to engage in cheating. There is, of course, no "standard size" for a community, and urban settings are likely to have a less clearly defined community size than suburban or rural ones. Charitable activities are easier to coordinate when the donors and recipients are mutually known. Barter arrangements can similarly be considered.

## QUESTION 34:

How can the performance and quality of hospitals and other organizations be assured?

## ANSWER:

Such responsibilities traditionally have been assigned to the Joint Commission on the Accreditation of Healthcare Organizations (JCAHO) and licensing committees of state and federal government. This approach has serious limitations, since there is insufficient incentive for the regulatory bodies to develop and promulgate practical quality measurements. Since they have no competition, JCAHO has been able to require hospitals to allocate resources in ways not always consistent with good management. No practical method of appeal is available to challenge JCAHO standards, however arbitrary they sometimes seem. Hospitals are thus effectively captive to a bureaucracy with negligible external controls. This bureaucracy then becomes vulnerable to the illusion that since it has largely unchecked power, it must then also have wisdom. One way to improve this might be for the federal government to certify one or more other accrediting bodies, so that hospitals would have a choice of quality consultants and accreditors. Competition would then provide incentives toward reasonableness.

## QUESTION 35:

How can patients assess the quality and reliability of the medical advice that they get?

## ANSWER:

One happy result of the technological revolution is the explosive expansion of available information. The Internet provides a huge resource of data, information, and sometimes even knowledge. Not all is of equal reliability, of course, but web sites managed by the National Institutes of Health, the National Library of Medicine, the Centers of Disease Control, the American Medical Association, and many others provide the patient-consumer with a vast array of practical advice. Patients can ask well-informed questions of their healthcare professionals and compare the answers with reliable standards.

## QUESTION 36:

Won't physicians object to the patients having access to the most up-to-date medical knowledge?

## ANSWER:

Good physicians won't object. One of the most proper and honored roles for physicians has been that of educator. Some, of course, will be uncomfortable with patients' informed questions, preferring to have his or her word accepted on the basis of authority alone. But physicians who welcome the opportunity to explain their thinking will find that their popularity increases, their advice is more valued, and the likelihood of lawsuits is reduced.

## QUESTION 37:

Isn't healthcare delivery analogous to a public utility?

## ANSWER:

The analogy isn't a very good one. Some similarities exist; equal access ought to be available to all. The quality of the product ought to be equal for all consumers, just as everyone should get the same quality of water or electricity. But beyond that, the analogy fails. Everyone needs the same kind of water or electricity. Everyone needs individualized medical care. Standard issue "one size fits all" works for many services and commodities, but quality medical care is neither of these. Uniformity makes the tasks of regulators and insurers easier, but as we have noted, they are only ancillary to the main task of healthcare. To see that everyone gets the same number of aspirin is not good care. To know who needs aspirin, how much, and when is what makes good care possible.

## QUESTION 38:

How can we be sure that professionals are competent?

## ANSWER:

There is no substitute for the well-informed judgment of the individual patient. Credentials such as specialty board certification are important, of course, as are recommendations from respected peers and colleagues. But in these judgments, as in so many areas of life, character is destiny. Does the professional caregiver treat you with courtesy and respect? Do you know that your concerns are heard, and as much as possible, thoughtfully considered, and explained? Does the advice make sense logically, and is it consistent with information gathered at reliable sources elsewhere? In other words, it is finally up to you to decide whose advice to believe, and it is idle to await a guarantee from organizations such as governments or insurance companies.

## QUESTION 39:

How is healthcare delivery likely to be organized a decade from now?

## ANSWER:

Citizens must make the final decisions. The current system of HMOs or "managed care" is structurally unsound, economically, politically, and morally. The incentive structure on which HMOs depend encourages rationing of care through deception. As this becomes clear to the large majority, we must search for better alternatives. There are two ways we can go—toward more governmental involvement or toward more individual responsibility. Our guess is that in ten years we will still be arguing this political question, but it is likely that a variety of experimental solutions will be tried. We think this will be all to the good.

## QUESTION 40:

With the system you advocate, what will happen when people change jobs or become temporarily unemployed?

## ANSWER:

Unlike most current plans that depend upon insurance, a community-based system with medical savings accounts as a major component would not be compromised by a change of jobs. The money in the account would be yours to use, and not dependent on the whims of bureaucrats and administrators. Catastrophic insurance, a necessary component especially for young people, would have to be continued by some means, of course, but a community-based system ought to provide for more options than now exist.

## QUESTION 41:

How should chronic mental illness be handled?

## ANSWER:

Modern advances in the scientific understanding of mental illness make it clear that there is no reason to segregate these problems from the rest of medicine. Chronic mental diseases are brain diseases, and most of the time treatable to the extent that major improvement is likely. Thus, the same system that treats strokes, mental retardation, and head injury can deal effectively with mental illness, without resort to prolonged hospitalization or other stigmatizing segregation. A medical care system should not promise to solve all the problems of human living. Elective or optional treatments for personality adjustment ought not, to our way of thinking, be a prominent feature of care. But that decision would be made by each individual using his own account.

## QUESTION 42:

How would you guard against the danger that people would elect to employ ineffective "alternative" treatments?

**ANSWER:**

We would not act as such guards. Judgment would be up to every individual. We think that, over time, experience would weed out less effective treatments without any regulations. As we see it, catastrophic insurance would be used only for treatments in the mainstream and scientifically sound. If someone wanted to use his or her medical savings account for an unproven treatment, that would be an individual choice. Such a choice has its hazards, of course, but we think the alternatives are worse. We never get tired of insisting that the only way to make a sound compromise with quality, availability, and cost is to return the responsibility for decisions on care to the individual patient.

**QUESTION 43:**

How would you deal with the problem of dropouts from a community-based plan?

**ANSWER:**

Individuals electing a style of care would be expected to have both a catastrophic coverage and a medical savings account, if employed. If the system we have described were to become the standard for the large majority, then medical savings accounts might become mandatory as payroll deductions.

**QUESTION 44:**

Why don't physicians police themselves?

**ANSWER:**

The simple answer is that physicians are not granted the legal power to do so, nor do we advocate that they should be. The modern world is simply too complex and interdependent to give any group such full autonomy. Would we wish lawyers, or politicians, or bakers to police themselves? Probably not. There are too many opportunities for a mediocre majority in any profession to use their putative "police" power to suppress honest and innovative competitors. We think the best form of policing has to do with an informed public making individual judgments. We believe also that state boards of registration serve a necessary function in investigating patterns of substandard practice, fraud, and other forms of abuse. One of the most important functions of such boards is to keep accurate and updated information on professionals which is available to the public.

## QUESTION 45:

Are there any other necessary services currently organized around the community?

## ANSWER:

There are some similarities in what we propose to fire fighting and fire prevention. We expect a firehouse in every community, funded through taxes or managed on a volunteer basis. We expect firefighters to advise us in safety matters. We know fire insurance is a necessity, but we usually don't set fires in order to collect it. This is analogous, of course, to catastrophic medical insurance. If there are many fires, we expect to pay the professionals. We don't expect our fire insurance to take care of paying for our fuel oil or to maintain our heating systems. Some houses are larger than others and their owners should pay more for insurance. The community passes ordinances that set minimum standards for fire safety. The analogy is, of course, not perfect for comparison with medical care, but it is close enough to allow us some creative thought in the matter.

## QUESTION 46:

Aren't there some flaws in the system you have described?

## ANSWER:

There certainly are. When one depends on the actions and responsibilities of many individuals, it is likely that there will be some disappointments. We have confidence that the political process will ensure that a reasonable safety net will emerge for whatever systems might be designed. In any case, we claim no omniscience in these matters. Our objective has been to take a fresh look at what has been an intractable political problem in America for too long. We believe we can build on the best emerging ideas, such as medical savings accounts with catastrophic insurance. We think any emerging system needs to be based on the best modern insights into the behavior of people in groups. But this is no utopia, and for that we make no apology.

## QUESTION 47:

Why have we not heard of this approach before?

**ANSWER:**

We wonder that too. We tried to rethink the problem of healthcare from scratch and build a construct covering all the necessary tasks. We tried to avoid the large set of encumbering and contradictory assumptions which have paralyzed us, and kept us in the habit of repeating the old arguments in a louder voice. Our approach may not have appeared before because it does not seem to accrue benefit to any of the usual special interests: government, corporations, or professionals. We tried to start from the perspective of the patient.

**QUESTION 48:**

You are the only ones who seem to be bringing forth some of these ideas. Shouldn't we wait for a consensus before we take you seriously?

**ANSWER:**

Many others have offered similar concepts. We hope we have put enough provocative ideas in one place so some of the murk and confusion about healthcare might be lifted. Some ideas can be both true and useful even if only a few people advance them.

**QUESTION 49:**

Won't your proposal favor the rich?

**ANSWER:**

Every practical system in human affairs can to some extent be construed to favor the rich or the well-connected. Medical care is no exception. Just as the rich will have more comfortable and safer housing, so will they always enjoy some advantage in this and every other service. But we argue that our plan provides a better system for all and that inequities are likely to be minimized by it. We see attempts to eliminate all inequality as a utopian illusion which would be likely to do much more harm than good. The real challenge is to find the practical solution that best elevates measures of health in a way consistent with freedom, democracy, and individual responsibility.

**QUESTION 50:**

Why did you write this book?

**ANSWER:**

For many years healthcare policy has been stalled in an unproductive debate. We asked why this might be, from a perspective of behavioral science. We then investigated the motives and incentives of the major actors. We tried to devise a method by which people could cooperate in the solution, rather than merely lobby for their own special interests. Like many of you, we are getting to the age when it is likely that we will fall into the clutches of the healthcare system soon; we hope the experience will be benign. And we were able to advance some of these ideas because we have reached a point in our careers where no amount of pressure or coercion by any special interest can cause us too much harm.

**QUESTION 51:**

Do you have an underlying philosophy that informs these conclusions?

**ANSWER:**

The history of Western philosophy has been, in essence, a debate between those who believe that the purpose of the individual is to serve the state and those who say the individual is the significant being and the state is a necessary, but ancillary, creation. We embrace the latter point of view.

# Glossary of Health Insurance Terms

**Adverse selection.** A situation in which people with more serious and costly illnesses apply for membership in particular health insurance plans, resulting in those plans having higher medical costs than groups that have healthier members.

**Allowable expenses.** The necessary, customary, and reasonable expenses that an insurer will cover.

**Alternative treatment plan.** Provision in managed care arrangements for treatment outside of a hospital.

**Ambulatory care.** Medical care provided on an out-patient (nonhospital) basis.

**Average length of stay.** Measure used by hospitals to determine the average number of days patients spend in their facilities. A managed care firm will often assign a length of stay to patients whey they enter a hospital and will monitor them to see that they don't exceed it.

**Capitation.** Method of payment for health services in which the insurer pays providers a fixed amount for each person served regardless of the type and number of services used. Some HMOs pay monthly capitation fees to doctors, often referred to as per-member, per-month amount.

**Case management.** A managed care technique in which a patient with a serious medical condition is assigned an individual who arranges for cost-effective treatment, often outside a hospital.

**Coinsurance or co-payment.** An amount a health insurance policy requires the insured to pay for medical and hospital service, after payment of a deductible.

**Community rating.** A method, based on geographical area, of calculating health insurance premiums for which employer groups and individuals pay the same rate.

**Concurrent review.** A managed care technique in which a representative of a managed care firm continuously reviews the charts of hospitalized patients to determine if they are staying too long and if the course of treatment is appropriate.

**Consolidated Omnibus Budget Reconciliation Act (COBRA).** Federal law that requires employers with more than 20 employees to extend group health insurance coverage for at least 18 months after employees leave their jobs. Employees must pay 102% of the premium.

**Cost containment.** An attempt to reduce the higher-than-necessary costs surrounding the allocation and consumption of healthcare. These costs may arise from inappropriately used services and from care that can be provided in less costly settings without harming the patient.

**Cost shifting.** A phenomenon occurring in the US healthcare system in which providers are reimbursed for their costs and subsequently raise their prices to other payers in an effort to recoup costs. Low reimbursement rates from government healthcare programs often cause providers to raise prices for medical care to private insurance carriers.

**Deductible.** An amount of covered expenses that must be paid by the insured before the insurance company begins to pay benefits.

**Diagnosis-related groups (DGRs).** A method of reimbursing providers based on the medical diagnosis for each patient. Hospitals receive a set amount determined in advance based on the length of time patients with a given diagnosis are likely to stay in the hospital. Also called prospective payment system.

**Employee Retirement Income Security Act (ERISA).** Federal law that establishes uniform standards for employer-sponsored benefit plans. Because of court decisions, law effectively prohibits states from experimenting with alternative health-financing arrangements without waivers from Congress.

**Exclusions.** Medical conditions specified in a policy for which the insurer will provide no benefits.

**Exclusive provider organization (EPO).** A healthcare payment and delivery arrangement in which members must obtain all their care from doctors and hospitals within an established network. If members go outside, no benefits are payable.

**Experience rating.** A method of calculating health insurance premiums for a group based entirely or partly on the risks the group presents. An employer whose employees are unhealthy will pay higher rates than another whose employees are healthier.

**Fee for service.** A method doctors use to charge for their services, setting their own fees for each service or procedure they perform.

**Fee schedule.** Maximum dollar amounts that are payable to healthcare providers. Medicare has a fee schedule for doctors who treat beneficiaries. Insurance companies have fee schedules that determine what they'll pay under the policies.

**First dollar coverage.** A health insurance policy with no required deductible.

**Gatekeeper.** Term given to a primary care physician in a managed care network who controls patient access to medical specialists.

**Gatekeeper PPO.** A healthcare payment and deliver system consisting of networks of doctors and hospitals. Members must choose a primary care physician, use doctors in the network, or face higher out-of-pocket costs.

**Health Insurance Purchasing Cooperative (HIPC).** A large group of employers and individuals functioning as an insurance broker to purchase health coverage, certify health plans, manage premiums and enrollment, and provide consumers with buying information. Also called health insurance purchasing group, health plan purchasing cooperative, and health insurance purchasing corporation.

**Health maintenance organization (HMO).** A healthcare payment and delivery system involving networks of doctors and hospitals.

**Hospital pre-authorization.** A managed care technique in which the insured obtains permission from a managed care organization before entering the hospital for nonemergency care.

**Hospital-surgical policy.** A type of health insurance policy that pays specific benefits for hospital services, including room-and-board surgery.

**Independent Practice Association (IPA).** An HMO in which doctors are usually paid fees for their services, and controls over services may be less stringent than in other types of HMOs.

**Long-term care.** A continuum of maintenance, custodial, and health services to the chronically ill, disabled, or retarded.

**Managed care.** A term that applies to the integration of healthcare delivery and financing. It includes arrangements with providers to supply healthcare services to members, criteria for the selection of healthcare providers, significant financial incentives for members to use providers in the plan, and formal programs to monitor the amount of care and quality of services.

**Managed competition.** A method for controlling healthcare costs by organizing employers, individuals, and other buyers of healthcare into large cooperatives that will purchase coverage for their members. Insurance companies and managed care organizations will compete to supply coverage for the lowest cost.

**Major medical policy.** A type of health insurance policy that provides benefits for most medical expenses, usually subject to a high maximum benefit, deductibles, and coinsurance.

**Mandated benefits.** Certain coverages, such as prenatal care, mammographic screening, and care for newborns that states require insurers to include in health insurance policies. Sometimes called state mandates.

**Medicaid.** A state–federal program that pays the healthcare bills for those people, regardless of age, who have insufficient income and assets to pay the costs themselves.

**Medicare.** Federal program under the Social Security Act that provides hospital and medical coverage to those 65 and older and to certain disabled individuals regardless of age.

**Medicare HMO.** A type of contract Medicare enters into with health maintenance organizations to provide benefits to HMO members. Members receiving benefits under this arrangement are "locked in"—that is, they must receive all their care from the HMO, or Medicare will not reimburse them.

**Medicare-supplement policy.** A type of health insurance policy that provides benefits for services Medicare does not cover.

**Open enrollment period.** Time during which uninsured employees may join a healthcare plan or insured employees can switch plans without proving they are healthy.

**Point of service.** A term that applies to certain health maintenance organizations and preferred provider organizations. Members in a point-of-service HMO or PPO can go outside the network for care, but their reimbursement will be less than if they had remained inside.

**Preexisting condition.** A physical or mental condition that an insured has prior to the effective date of coverage. Policies may exclude coverage for such conditions for a specified period of time.

**Preferred Provider Organization (PPO).** A healthcare payment and delivery system with networks of doctors and hospitals. System may place looser restrictions on doctors than HMOs. Members are not always required to choose a primary care physician and can go outside the network for care, but they receive lower reimbursement.

**Preferred risks.** People with few, if any, medical problems whom insurance companies like to insure because they present little likelihood of filing claims in the near future.

**Prepaid Health Care Act.** Federal law passed in 1973 that sets standards for federally qualified health maintenance organizations. Among the standards are minimum benefits and provision for grievance procedures.

**Primary care.** Basic care including initial diagnosis and treatment, preventive services, maintenance of chronic conditions, and referral to specialists.

**Primary care physician.** Physician in a managed care network who supervises medical care for members and makes referrals to specialists, if needed.

**Rationing.** The allocation of medical care by price or availability of services.

**Second opinion review.** A managed care technique in which a second physician is consulted regarding diagnosis or course of treatment. Thought to be of questionable effectiveness in reducing costs.

**Shadow pricing.** Tendency of health insurers to price their services at the same or nearly the same level as indemnity insurance plans.

**Usual, customary, and reasonable (UCR).** Amounts charged by healthcare providers that are consistent with charges for similar providers for the same or nearly the same services in a given area.

**Utilization.** Patterns of usage for a particular medical service such as hospital care or physician visits.

**Utilization review.** A managed care technique in which the managed care firm or insurance company attempts to reduce the length of hospital stays and the number of unnecessary hospital admissions.

**Waiver.** A provision in a health insurance policy in which specific medical conditions a person already has are excluded from coverage.

## NOTE

We thank the *Los Angeles Times* for permission to reprint this glossary.

# Annotated Bibliography

Burt, R. S. *Toward a Structural Theory of Action*. New York: Academic Press, 1982. This is a classic source on network models of social structure, perception, and action. Of particular interest is the author's view of the inherent division of labor that underlies social structure.

Ellickson, R. C. *Order without Law—How Neighbors Settle Disputes*. Cambridge, MA: Harvard University Press, 1991. A classic study about how neighbors can solve disputes without recourse to legal means.

Fisher, C. S. *To Dwell Among Friends*. Chicago: University of Chicago Press, 1982. The author documents different types of personal networks and how behavior and trust differ as a function of network type. Of particular interest is the author's discussion of whether the decline in community perspective leads to a weakening of social bonds and psychological and social disorganization.

Gruter, M., and Masters, R. D. (eds.). *Ostracism: A Social and Biological Phenomenon*. New York: Elsevier, 1986. This is still the most complete book dealing with the psychological and physiological consequences of social ostracism and how these consequences influence cooperative behavior.

Hanson, V. D., and Heath, J. *The Demise of Classical Education and the Recovery of Greek Wisdom*. New York: The Free Press, 1998. The authors outline how the ancient Greeks were responsible for our present Western notions of constitutional government, free speech, individual rights, civilian control of the military, separation between religious and political authority, middle-class egalitarianism, private property, and free scientific inquiry.

Illich, I. *Medical Nemesis*. New York: Pantheon, 1976. Illich not only argues that the medical establishment has become a major threat to health but also that we need to redefine our concept of health as well as the kind of civilization that produces the type of health we have. This book is essential reading for discussions dealing with the underpinnings of healthcare.

Kaufman, H. *Time, Chance, and Organizations* (2nd ed.). Chatham, NJ: Chatham

House, 1991. The author outlines his theory of organizational survival and demise, and in the process takes the discourse of organizational behavior to new levels of insight and complexity. The book is particularly applicable to the current plight of HMOs.

McGuire, M. T., and Troisi, A. *Darwinian Psychiatry*. New York: Oxford University Press, 1998. The authors discuss in detail many of the concepts found in Chapters 8 and 9.

McKenzie, N. F. (ed.). *Beyond Crisis*. New York: Meridian, 1994. This is the source of many of the statistics developed in Chapter 4.

Mendelsohn, R. S. *Confessions of a Medical Heretic*. Chicago: Contemporary Books, 1979. The author argues that approximately 2.4 million unnecessary operations are performed every year in the United States and that these operations cost about 12,000 lives. Whether this figure has increased or decreased in recent years is uncertain.

Rose, S. *Biology Beyond Determinism*. New York: Oxford University Press, 1998. This book addresses many of the complexities of human biology, with particular emphasis on areas in which we know little to practically nothing. The book is sobering with respect to the possibility of eliminating or even controlling disease in the near future.

Starr, P. *The Social Transformation of American Medicine*. New York: Basic Books, 1982. The author documents the rise of a sovereign profession and the making of a vast industry.

Starr, P. *The Logic of Health Care Reform*. New York: Whittle Books, 1994. The author outlines how the Clinton healthcare plan would work. His key point is that the plan represents input from all parts of healthcare. The model he advocates may work well enough when dealing with political compromise but differs significantly from many of the arguments presented here.

Stevens, R. *In Sickness and in Wealth*. New York: Basic Books, 1989. The author documents how American hospitals are unique and represent a combination of public and private institutions that are at once charities and businesses, social welfare institutions and icons of US sciences, wealth, and technical achievement. This multiplicity of roles and purposes is a major contributor to the crisis they face today.

Walton, M. *The Deming Management Method*. New York: Perigee Books, 1986. The author summarizes the work of management consultant W. Edwards Deming in practical form.

Wilson, E. O. *Sociobiology*. Cambridge MA: Harvard University Press, 1975. This work is arguably the single most important book of this century dealing with the evolution of behavior.

# Index

## About the Authors

MICHAEL T. McGUIRE is Professor of Psychiatry, UCLA School of Medicine, a member of the Brain Research Institute, and Director of the Sepulveda Veterans Administration/UCLA Nonhuman Primate Laboratory. He is the author or coauthor of more than 150 journal articles and four books, including *Darwinian Psychiatry* (1998) with Alfonso Troisi.

WILLIAM H. ANDERSON is Lecturer at the Harvard Medical School and Senior Psychiatrist, Massachusetts General Hospital. In addition to having held a variety of teaching and administrative positions, he is the author of more than 70 articles in scientific and policy journals.